'*The Gambling Establishment* is in part a metaphor for the transformation of modern gambling into an anti-democratic process that transfers wealth from the poor to the rich. By virtue of its ability to engender behavioural addiction, modern gambling has become the moral equivalent of the tobacco industry. The good news is that the pendulum is beginning to swing back to a place where society and its most vulnerable members are at least being given a fair chance. Jim Orford's masterful exposé of the *Gambling Establishment* provides an agenda of remedial proposals not only for the deplorable British gambling situation but also for the problems faced by other countries as well.'

– **Thomas F. Babor**, Professor of Community Medicine and
Public Health, University of Connecticut School of Medicine,
Farmington, CT, USA

'This vital book is a rallying cry for change in how governments regulate gambling. It outlines in forensic detail the ways in which a powerful industry has exploited regulatory loopholes for unsustainable commercial gain. Orford lays bare the techniques of deception and marketing that have served the industry's quest for limitless profit, and shows how unbridled gambling has damaged the lives of individuals, communities and the wider economy. This is a timely and determined book: it is a manifesto for radical change, and strengthens the case for a new British Gambling Act.'

– **Tom Watson**, MP, Deputy Leader of the British Labour Party and
Shadow Secretary of State for Digital, Culture, Media and Sport

'A fascinating window on the world of commercial gambling, *The Gambling Establishment* comprehensively undoes the official narrative that gambling is good, clean fun and shows instead that it is both addictive and a threat to public health. Anyone wishing to understand how gambling has become so prevalent in our society must read this important book, which should be compulsory reading for all ministers and politicians.'

– **Rebecca Cassidy**, Professor of Anthropology, Goldsmiths,
University of London

'That Jim's ideas on the regulation of gambling are no longer peripheral but now mainstream is testament to the strength of his philosophy. Where his voice was once marginalised, it is now the ideological centre of gravity. This intellectual paradigm shift away from locating blame with individuals and onto harmful products provided the justification for restrictions on Fixed Odds Betting Terminals, and this book acts as a compelling manual for navigating this new context, particularly preparing for a potential backlash from the Gambling Establishment.'

– **Matt Zarb–Cousin**, Spokesperson for the Stop the FOBTs campaign

'This is a comprehensive account of Big Gambling as it has become established in Britain and globally in recent decades, which details the social and health problems it has brought. Orford unmasks the deception about chances of winning often built into gambling machines and procedures. He dissects the arguments gambling interests and government agencies use to justify the new status quo. This is a thoughtful and comprehensive book presenting a compelling case for change.'
– **Robin Room**, Professor, La Trobe University, Australia and Stockholm University, Sweden

'When we set up Gambling with Lives in 2018, Jim Orford was the first name that people mentioned when we wanted to know about gambling research. When we met we understood why he was so highly regarded: his knowledge was vast and in depth . . . and he was truly independent. More than that, he had personal experience of the impact that gambling addiction could have on individuals and families. Jim understood. His narrative and reflections on gambling are essential reading for anyone involved in wanting to tackle the harms that gambling does.'
– **Liz and Charles Ritchie**, Co-chairs of Gambling with Lives

'Professor Orford continues to clearly raise the issues and need for reform in the gambling industry. This is a much needed and timely contribution which reinforces the urgent need for change as the UK edges towards the lip of a gambling epidemic.'
– **Lord Chadlington**, Conservative Peer

THE GAMBLING ESTABLISHMENT

There are now signs that, after decades of phenomenal growth, the era of unrestrained gambling liberalisation may be coming to an end. However, the power of the *Gambling Establishment* is formidable, and it will certainly fight back. Drawing on research and policy examples from around the world, the book provides a unified understanding of the dangerousness of modern commercialised gambling, how its expansion has been deliberately or inadvertently supported, and how the backlash is now occurring.

The term *Gambling Establishment* is defined to include the industry which sells gambling, governments which support it, and a wider network of organisations and individuals who have subscribed to the 'responsible gambling' Establishment discourse. Topics covered include the psychology of how gambling is now being advertised and promoted and the way it is designed to deceive gamblers about their chances of winning; the increased exposure of young people to gambling and the alignment of gambling with sport; understanding the experience of gambling addiction; the various public health harms of gambling at individual, family, community and societal levels; and how evidence has been used to resist change. The book's final chapter offers the author's manifesto for policy change, designed with Britain particularly in mind but likely to have relevance elsewhere.

With detailed examples given of the ways a number of countries are responding to these threats to their citizens' health, this book will be of global interest for academics, researchers, policymakers and service providers in the field of gambling or other addictions specifically, and public health and social policy generally.

Jim Orford is a long-standing, internationally recognised researcher and writer in the fields of addiction and community psychology, one of the UK's leading academics on the subject of gambling, and well-known for his critical views on policy. In 2012 he set up the Gambling Watch UK website to help campaign for a public health approach to gambling.

THE GAMBLING ESTABLISHMENT

Challenging the Power of the Modern Gambling Industry and its Allies

Jim Orford

Routledge
Taylor & Francis Group

LONDON AND NEW YORK

First published 2020
by Routledge
2 Park Square, Milton Park, Abingdon, Oxon OX14 4RN

and by Routledge
52 Vanderbilt Avenue, New York, NY 10017

Routledge is an imprint of the Taylor & Francis Group, an informa business

British Library Cataloguing-in-Publication Data
A catalogue record for this book is available from the British Library

Library of Congress Cataloging-in-Publication Data
A catalog record for this book has been requested

ISBN: 978-0-367-08568-1 (hbk)
ISBN: 978-0-367-08570-4 (pbk)
ISBN: 978-0-367-08571-1 (ebk)

Typeset in Bembo
by Apex CoVantage, LLC

CONTENTS

List of Tables   ix
List of Figures   x

Introduction   1

1   The new backlash against the growth of commercial gambling   5

2   The Gambling Establishment: The industry and its allies
    inside and outside government   26

3   The establishment discourse: Five ways we were told how to
    think about gambling   42

4   How gambling is forcibly advertised and sold in the modern era   58

5   Is modern gambling fraudulent? How players are deceived
    about the chances of winning   73

6   Understanding gambling addiction: Bringing personal
    experience and theory together   90

7   Gambling's harm to individuals, families, communities,
    and society   109

8   How the Gambling Establishment has used evidence to
     support its position   128

9   Resisting the power of the Gambling Establishment:
     A manifesto for change   142

References   *167*
Index   *183*

TABLES

1.1   Twenty-first century examples of countries that have taken decisions to reduce the numbers or dangerousness of electronic gambling machines (EGMs)   7

1.2   Examples of actions being taken by countries in an effort to control online gambling   13

2.1   Size of public revenue from gambling in a number of countries (estimates in Sulkunen *et al.*, 2019, pp 150–1)   36

4.1   Some of the main conclusions to be drawn from studies of how gambling is advertised   71

7.1   A summary of some of the main areas of gambling's harm   111

9.1   A manifesto for how gambling should be better managed in Britain (and elsewhere) in the 2020s and 2030s   143

FIGURES

2.1   The British Gambling Establishment   40
3.1   Five elements of the Gambling Establishment discourse   44
5.1   Examples of apparent and actual percent return to player (RTP) for
      EGM and online sports betting (EGMs with relatively low and
      high RTP, Harrigan & Dixon, 2010; Online outcome and in-play
      betting, LaBrie *et al.*, 2007)   82

INTRODUCTION

My previous book on this subject, *An Unsafe Bet*, was published in 2011 and was subtitled *The Dangerous Rise of Gambling and the Debate We Should Be Having*. That was at a time when the extraordinary growth of gambling, and the complacent thinking that went with it, were rampant and apparently unstoppable. Those of us in the health field who thought we saw the dangers were not hopeful of a change of direction. The climate in which I am completing the present book is different. In Britain there are signs that the tide may be turning. The Conservative Government has been persuaded, against industry advice, to make a substantial change to what has been the most profitable type of electronic gambling machine. The Labour Party has called for more sweeping changes and for a completely new Gambling Act to replace the 2005 Act which rendered Britain one of Europe's most liberal gambling regimes. The era of unrestrained gambling liberalisation in Britain, and perhaps elsewhere, may be coming to an end. Citizens are beginning to find their voice. The backlash is under way. However, the power of what I shall call the *Gambling Establishment* – the gambling industry and its allies inside and outside governments – is formidable, and it will certainly fight back.

The first chapter of the present book provides more detail about the new counterreaction to dangerous gambling in Britain and elsewhere. It looks at the concerns being expressed about modern machine gambling and the uncontrolled spread of online gambling, as well as the spread of casinos, and the ways in which a number of countries are responding to these threats to their citizens' health. The particular dangers of online gambling for young people, and the grey area between social media and gambling, are discussed.

Chapter 2 introduces the expression the *Gambling Establishment* to refer to a powerful alliance of interests which collectively has been responsible for the modern growth in gambling and therefore for the harm it is causing. The *Gambling*

Establishment includes not only the industry which sells gambling and governments which support it but also a range of non-government organisations and other allies which knowingly or inadvertently support liberalisation and oppose further regulation of gambling. That wider network includes financial, advertising, academic and service-providing organisations and individuals who have been drawn into the web of dependencies on gambling or who have been taken in by Establishment rhetoric about the place of modern commercial gambling in society.

Establishment thinking about gambling – the official gambling discourse – was utterly transformed in the modern era of liberalised gambling. No longer was gambling to be seen as immoral, irrational, exploitative, a vice that a nation should be ashamed of. Chapter 3 examines five key elements of the Establishment discourse. Alongside the selling of their products the gambling industry sold the ideas that their businesses were no different from any others, that the commodities they dealt in were not only harmless if used properly but were positively beneficial for individuals and communities, that the freedom of citizens to use their products as they choose is a fundamental right not to be interfered with, and, perhaps most important of all, that those who do experience difficulty using these commodities are failing to show due responsibility. There are encouraging signs that the popularity of the personal-responsibility discourse may be waning.

Chapters 4 and 5 focus on the psychology of how, in the modern era of gambling liberalisation, gambling is advertised and promoted (Chapter 4) and is designed in such a way that gamblers are continually being deceived about their chances of winning (Chapter 5). Two general conclusions about modern gambling promotion are highlighted. One is the increased exposure of children and young people to gambling advertising. The other is how gambling is promoted in ways which not only use all the tricks of the advertising trade but which also try to give a false impression of what engaging in modern forms of gambling really entails – depicting gambling as a low-risk/high-control pastime, full of fun, with a good prospect of winning money. The reality – a high likelihood of losing money and the danger of addiction – is concealed. The research reviewed from a number of countries concerning how modern gambling is structured shows, amongst other things, how volatility disguises the operator's advantage, why information about payback percentage is misleading, the importance of skewed distributions of wins, and other ways gamblers are being seduced into spending more, such as near misses, complex and in-play bets, and the illusion of skill and control. The concept of 'losses disguised as wins', introduced through Canadian research on machine gambling, throws light on the deceptiveness of modern commercial gambling of any type.

Chapters 6 and 7 take two complementary approaches to the dangers of gambling: the addiction and public health 'harms' approaches, respectively. It is argued that gambling addiction is now not only well established as a recognised form of addiction but can claim to be one of the clearest forms, even a prototype case, of addiction. A substantial part of Chapter 6 is devoted to extracts from book-length or qualitative research first-person accounts. Five characteristics emerge as central to the intensely emotional experience of being addicted to gambling – preoccupation, distorted thinking, secrecy, personality change and feelings of divided self. The chapter proceeds to summarise my understanding about the fundamental nature of addiction, of which gambling addiction is a prime example. Addiction is explained as a strong, entrenched and seriously harmful habit. Studies of the neuroscience of addiction support that model.

Chapter 7 looks in some detail at the various individual, family, community and societal harms of gambling which have been identified. In summary it is argued that the acceptance of gambling in its present forms as a normal part of society threatens that society's well-being in a number of ways: by adversely affecting ill-health, homelessness and crime statistics, threatening family life, diminishing the vibrancy of town centres, contributing to inequality, and adding to the risks faced by the young. In the process it may be a contributor to an undermining of some of a society's positive traditional values.

Chapter 8 looks critically at the way the *Gambling Establishment* uses evidence to bolster its support for the continued expansion of commercial gambling. It is shown how the process of gathering evidence about gambling and the harm that it may be doing is being unduly influenced by the gambling-providing industry and its supporters. Two British examples are used as illustrations: a research pro-gramme on gambling machines in betting shops; and the way evidence has been interpreted to resist calls for controls on TV gambling advertising and sports spon-sorship. Giving the false impression that evidence is being used objectively serves to consolidate the *Gambling Establishment's* powerful position.

The final chapter provides my manifesto for change. A number of proposals for the way forward are outlined. They are designed with the British gambling con-text in mind but are likely to have relevance elsewhere. They fall into four areas. The first, and most important, is a fundamental rethinking of the basic approach to gambling regulation. That would mean: a comprehensive new Gambling Act; the replacement of the ordinary business/responsible gambling ideology with an alternative dangerous consumption/public health perspective; a proper national strategy for gambling produced by Government; the Health Ministry to play a leading role; and gambling harm prevention, treatment and research, funded out of general taxation, to be administered by a new body completely independent of the industry or regulator.

Second, the issue of gambling advertising needs to be reconsidered, with the protection of children and young people as a primary consideration, including a proper pre-watershed ban on television advertising and a ban on gambling company sponsorship of football and other sporting teams. Third, harm reduction policies should be rethought, shifting the emphasis away from reliance on ineffective forms of HR such as education and identifying problem players towards HR measures of sufficient scope and magnitude, including a minimum age of 18 years for all gambling, clearer adherence to the principle of preventing ambient gambling, and some combination of absolute and mandatory-self-chosen loss- and time-limit setting, which render gambling products less dangerous. Last, but by no means least, there is need for a proper comprehensive National Health Service–based system of treatment for people with gambling problems and help for affected families.

Jim Orford

March 2019

1

THE NEW BACKLASH AGAINST THE GROWTH OF COMMERCIAL GAMBLING

In Poland in 2009 several very senior politicians, including the Deputy Prime Minister and Ministers for Sport and for Justice, resigned over the issue. In 2010 the Australian federal Government nearly fell because of it. And in 2018 the UK's Minister for Sport resigned for the same reason. What was the issue that had become so political in those three very different countries and in so many others too? The answer is gambling. More accurately, the failure of governments to protect their citizens from the late 20th and early 21st centuries' expansion of commercial gambling.

Gambling is now no longer gambling as we once knew it. The many ways in which gambling can be offered online and the much more sophisticated and high-powered gambling machines – both taking full advantage of technological changes – are among the most obvious ways in which gambling has been transformed in a remarkably short period of time. The much greater diversity of sports betting, the opportunity to gamble on numerous events 24 hours a day, the constant advertisements and inducements to gamble, the greater size of lottery and bingo jackpots, and the rise of betting exchanges, spread betting and personal 'trading' are amongst other features of this changed world of gambling. Country after country, jurisdiction after jurisdiction, has been seduced by the money to be made.

The drive for this expansion and transformation has come from the profit-making industry itself and from governments which have put financial gain first and made protection of the public a lower priority. The public's view has not often been heard, and when occasionally it has been heard it is overruled by the powerful forces of what now amounts to a *Gambling Establishment*. In the words of one academic colleague, from New Zealand, 'gambling has moved from being a dispersed cottage industry to a high-volume consumer enterprise – an industrial revolution on a worldwide scale' (Adams, 2016).

If one examines how this transformation came about, one thing that stands out is the opposition to the expansion of gambling which was always evident and which had to be overcome. Gambling has always been controversial. Citizens, and frequently their leaders, have always been aware of the harm that gambling can cause. A number of witnesses to gambling in the final decades of the 20th century predicted a counteraction to growing liberalisation. One went so far as to say, of gambling in the USA, 'The 1990s and the first decade of the 21st century will be the final boom. By 2029 it will be outlawed, again' (Rose, 1991). If that is what he hoped for, he was perhaps over-optimistic, but of signs of a backlash there are now plenty from around the world.

I will begin by looking at the backlash against machine gambling, illustrating the point by reference to a number of specific countries. I will go on to look at the concerns being expressed about online gambling, particularly concerns about effects for children and young people, and the ways in which a number of countries are responding. After then considering reactions to the spread of casinos globally, I will describe the reaction against liberalised gambling which is now growing in my own country, Britain.[1]

The backlash against the new generation of high-powered dangerous gambling machines

Behind the extraordinary rise in gambling internationally in just a few decades lies the ingenuity of a diverse industry whose main interest, naturally enough, is to make as much money as possible. Nowhere is this clearer than in the case of the EGMs, the electronic gambling machines. They were already seen as troublesome in Britain years ago in the first half of the 20th century. The Lord Chief Justice in 1927 described the slot machine as 'a pest and a most mischievous pest', and after World War II, the 1951 Royal Commission on Betting, Lotteries and Gaming, despite its more relaxed approach to gambling compared to earlier such reports, recommended that gaming machines should be illegal (Dixon, 1991). Similarly, the foresightful Royal Commission into Gambling in Western Australia in 1974 recommended sticking to the policy of confining gambling machines to casinos on the grounds that they required no skill or social contact and appeared to be addictive.

Little could those who made such statements years ago have anticipated the changes that would be made to EGMs in years to come. The seductive features of gambling machines of that time now look trivial compared to more recent developments. Long gone are the mechanical one-armed bandits of yesteryear, now replaced by complex electronic devices offering endless permutations of betting choices accompanied by attractive state-of-the-art visual and auditory displays. Later, in Chapter 5, we shall examine more closely the addiction potential of these dangerous inventions.

An important international review appeared in 2019 from a group of prominent experts in the field of public health whose previous summaries of international research on alcohol, for example, have been highly influential. That this group should turn its focus on gambling is itself an indication of the increased critical attention now being devoted to the subject of gambling worldwide. About EGMs they say, 'EGMs generate much, if not most of the profit for the gambling industry, and most of the harm caused by it' (Sulkunen *et al.*, 2019). They point out that even casinos make most of their profit from EGMs.

Table 1.1 shows examples of countries that have taken decisions to try and reverse the trend towards increasing numbers of dangerous EGMs in accessible public areas such as bars and cafes in several European countries and pubs and clubs in Australia – what has been called 'suburban gambling' in Australia and 'ambient gambling' in the UK. Several points about the backlash in those countries are telling and help inform us about the way forward in other places including Britain.

One thing to note is that resistance has often been keenest at the local level. In Italy the lead was largely taken by an increasing number of municipalities and regions, often opposed by the national Government. For example, the Piedmont Region passed a law in 2016 that slot machines could not be placed less than 500 metres away from schools, places of worship, shops that buy gold, therapeutic communities and cash machines. In the Czech Republic, where the law governing gambling allows individual municipalities regulatory control over the availability of EGMs

TABLE 1.1 Twenty-first century examples of countries that have taken decisions to reduce the numbers or dangerousness of electronic gambling machines (EGMs)

Norway[1]	EGMs brought under state monopoly in 2003; after unsuccessful court challenges, all EGMs removed in 2007; safer machines, including setting session loss limits, reintroduced from 2009
Italy[2]	Agreement in 2017 to halve the number of gambling venues nationally, including bars and tobacco shops, by the end of 2019, and to reduce the number of EGMs by 35%
Poland[3]	Gambling Law of 2009 brought in tighter regulation of gambling including availability, advertising, operation of games and taxation: number of gambling venues dropped by half in the next year and low prize EGMs eliminated by 2015
Australia[4]	In 2010 Government agreed EGM reform to include mandatory setting of individual loss limits; Government backtracks after industry campaigning against the reform
Czech Republic[5]	In 2017 Government issued guidelines for the imposition of mandatory limits for players' losses, requiring online and land-based operators to set maximum hourly loss limits
Russia[6]	In 2006 a law passed to confine legal gambling, other than a limited number of bookmakers, betting shops and charity lotteries, to four 'gambling zones', each to be located at a distance from major cities

[1] Borch (2018); [2] Rolando & Scavarda (2018); [3] Wieczorek & Bujalski (2018); [4] Adams (2016); [5] Casino Players Report (2017); [6] Vasiliev & Bernhard (2012).

in their areas, and even allows them to ban machines altogether, it was reported that the option to ban machines had been taken up in more than 200 towns and villages in the Republic, and several hundred other municipalities had regulated availability, sometimes through local referenda. In Norway, too, individual cities and regions were reported to be vying at one time to be among the first to ban EGMs altogether. Also very influential have been grassroots movements. Examples are: the No Slot Movement in Italy, which includes lay and Catholic non-profit organisations and individual citizens; and several non-government organisations in the Czech Republic such as Citizens Against Gambling led by activists and ex-gamblers, and one in Norway led by Lill-Tove Bergmo whose husband was recovering from problem gambling (Borch, 2018; Rolando & Scavarda, 2018; Szczyrba *et al.*, 2015).

Press reaction to evidence of growing gambling harm has played an important role, for example in provoking the Norwegian Government's uniquely strong response (Borch, 2018). The press there had been increasingly critical of national gambling policy after the operation of machine gambling was opened up to humanitarian and sports organisations and commercial operators in the 1990s. In Russia, also, the change in the law followed negative media coverage of the Russian gambling industry in 2006 (Vasiliev & Bernhard, 2012).

Another point to note is the resistance such movements meet, not just from the gambling industry, but also from governments slow to institute reform. Change in Italy only occurred after lengthy negotiations with a recalcitrant national Government and in Norway only after a legal battle with the EGMs Operators' Association. In a number of countries, a political crisis ensued in the process. In Poland, there was serious political fallout from the gambling controversy, with several Ministers resigning, accused of involvement in unofficial lobbying and serving the vested interests of the gambling industry. In Australia, Prime Minister Kevin Rudd was already on record as saying in 2007, 'I hate pokie machines', and a few years later, following a national election that produced a hung parliament, Prime Minister Julia Gillard struck a bargain with an independent MP whose support was conditional on Government agreement to bring in mandatory pre-commitment (i.e. requiring machine gamblers to pre-set a maximum loss limit: see Chapter 9). Seeing the threat to industry interests, ClubsNSW committed up to A$40 million to oppose the reform, which funded, amongst other things, an advertising campaign entitled 'It's UN-Australian'. In the event, Gillard caved in to the pressure, including pressure from her own back-benchers, survived by gaining parliamentary support elsewhere, and adopted the weak alternative of slowly introducing a system of *voluntary* pre-commitment (Adams, 2016). In Britain, the resignation of Sports Minister Tracey Crouch in November 2018 influenced Government to relent and reduce a delay in implementing an already long-delayed decision to reduce the maximum allowed stake size on the fixed-odds type of EGMs in betting shops (more about the FOBTs later), thus forcing the Chancellor of the Exchequer to go back on a budget announcement made only a few days previously.

It is also important to note straight away that different jurisdictions do things very differently when it comes to gambling (see Chapter 2). It comes as a surprise to those who have got used to the proliferation of EGMs in easily accessible venues in their own countries, that EGMs remain illegal outside casinos in France and also in the state of Western Australia, both public gambling machine-free oases in continents that have otherwise ignored the warnings about the dangers (Bruneau et al., 2017; Marionneau & Berret, 2018).

Resistance to the uncontrolled spread of online gambling

Machine gambling figures large in the present book, but the inexorable rise of gambling has been a general phenomenon and by no means confined to one type of gambling. The other form of gambling which will crop up repeatedly is gambling online, or 'internet gambling', as it is often called. What used to be referred to as 'remote gambling' began not so very long ago when it became possible to place bets over the telephone. But since then the internet has changed everything, creating a situation in which gambling is available 24 hours a day without the need to enter a gambling venue. The first time the general public was able to gamble online is said to have been in 1995 when the International Lottery in Liechtenstein allowed lottery tickets to be purchased online (Williams et al., 2012). New companies emerged which had no 'land-based' gambling venues, provoking established gambling operators to expand their range of products to include online gambling. The number of online gambling sites has increased at a staggering rate year by year, from a mere handful or two in the mid-1990s to several thousands by 2010 (Banks, 2014). By then there were gambling companies operating out of over 50 different territorial jurisdictions, among the most important being Malta, Netherlands Antilles, the Kahnawake Mohawk Territory in North America, Gibraltar and the United Kingdom.

It is worth pointing out here that the internet not only makes it possible to provide, in online or virtual mode, forms of gambling such as sports betting, poker tournaments or casino games which are already familiar in land-based form. It also stimulated, and continues to give rise to, new forms and modes of gambling. Early examples included spread betting, with its origins in stock market trading, and the use of 'betting exchanges' where a betting intermediary such as the company Betfair brokers bets between individuals – the commercialisation of what used to be an agreement to gamble made privately by individuals without the need for a commercial intermediary. These two, still quite new, ways of gambling provide yet further illustrations of how gambling has changed and expanded in ways that make it more commercial, more global and almost certainly more dangerous.

Spread betting is particularly dangerous because, depending upon how far the result – for example the price of gold, the rise or fall of the Dow Jones or FTSE100 stock market index or the number of runs England makes against Australia in a cricket match – deviates from what is predicted and bet on, the amount lost may much exceed the original stake. At the same time it illustrates the growing fuzzy area between traditional gambling, such as betting on the outcome of a horse race, and the increasingly well-recognised 'gambling' facet of financial trading.

Another newish development gaining popularity around the world, particularly in the USA, where the Unlawful Internet Gambling Enforcement Act (UIGEA) has prohibited online sports betting across state borders (Matuszewski, 2014), is 'fantasy sports betting' in which people make bets on imaginary teams consisting of real players. Meanwhile, as we shall see, an aspect of the multi-faceted modern gambling world that is stimulating as much concern and opposition as any is the fast-growing, murky grey area between social media and gambling.

The dangers of online gambling for young people

The world has become an ever more dangerous place for young people where gambling is concerned. Indeed, it has become more dangerous for us all – which is a principal argument of this book. Mark Griffiths (e.g. 2010), a psychologist and internationally acknowledged British expert on adolescent gambling who has worked with the gambling industry and is by no means an all-out critic of gambling liberalisation, has warned about the dangers of online gambling for young people. He has made several good points about this. Online gambling, he says, because of the technology involved, poses a particular risk for young people because it so closely resembles video games, is likely to be confused with them, and is seen as fun rather than as gambling. Ideas of skill and luck are likely to be confused by children when gambling is presented in the context of a predominantly skill-based game. Gambling may become 'normalised' as a legitimate activity that children and adolescents can engage in rather than it being seen as an adult leisure activity. Children and adolescents may be conditioned towards holding unrealistic notions and positive attitudes towards gambling.

Another international expert who has warned about the dangers of online gambling for young people is Sally Gainsbury (2012) of Southern Cross University, Australia, who carried out a review of what was then known about internet gambling. She pointed out that online gambling was more heavily concentrated amongst younger adults than was the case for other forms of gambling. Furthermore, the evidence was that engagement in online gambling was more strongly associated with problem gambling than engagement in non-online forms of gambling. She concluded that few sites had reliable measures for assessing players' ages and identities, and hence age verification was not sufficiently effective in preventing underage play. A complication was that many online sites offered 'practice' or 'free play' games, typically with no age restrictions but often linked to real money sites or games and assumed by many to be a way of training future customers. The British gambling regulator, the Gambling Commission (GC), has regularly carried out 'test purchasing' to check whether gambling providers attempt to verify players' ages, and how effectively they do it. It was still in 2019 calling for improvements (Gambling Commission, 2019a).

A further concern, Gainsbury's review pointed out, was the variety of ways in which online gambling could be conducted and the likelihood that this would change rapidly in the future in a way that was difficult to predict. Although the large majority of online gambling might at that time have been conducted through personal computers connected to the internet, online operators were busy developing gambling opportunities for other platforms, including mobile gambling undertaken on remote wirelessly connected devices, interactive television and gaming consoles. A mere five years later such warnings already seemed outdated. One of the most alarming developments since that review was written, of great concern to parents and carers and increasingly to governments and their gambling regulators, has been the growing link between gambling and sports popular among children and young people. Researchers, particularly in Australia and in Britain, have explored the ways in which the marketing of betting has become embedded within sport and how it appeals to fan loyalty, with gambling products linked to professional sporting teams, professional players and other celebrities. We shall return to look at this in more detail in Chapter 4.

The grey area between social media and gambling

The convergence of gambling with digital media and the rapid pace of development of new technologies, often quickly superseded by new ones, has led to the point where there is now confusion about what is gambling and what is not. That has made it difficult to identify all those who are in effect providing gambling of the kind that may be especially attractive to adolescents and children. Already in 2009 a prescient paper was describing in some detail a number of forms of internet activity that fall into this grey area, warning that they 'may be problematic for adolescents because they promote positive attitudes towards gambling, portray gambling in glamorised and/or misrepresentative ways, and . . . are freely available and playable by adolescents and children' (King *et al.*, 2009).

The first such category was online games in which a player can win or lose points that can be transferred into real money. *Project Entropia* and *World of Warcraft* were examples. It was especially difficult to know whether or not a game should be classified as 'gambling' when it mixed skill and chance. Whilst such games might largely be skill-based, subscriptions enabled the player to win jackpots, prizes and awards at random intervals, and furthermore some online games featured advertisements and direct links to online gambling sites.

Only a few years later, in 2017, the expression 'loot boxes' – otherwise known as 'crates', 'chests', 'bundles' or 'cases' – had been coined, and they were hitting the news around the world. Gambling regulators had cottoned on to the threat posed by awarding game players random digital items in purchasable 'loot crates', and governments from Sweden, France and Belgium to Australia were asking how they should be controlled (Ars Technica, 2018; The Conversation, 2018; The Guardian, 2018a). *Star Wars: Battlefront II* was just one of many games caught up in the controversy, but sports type games such as *FIFA Ultimate Team* and

Forza Motorsport 7 were others that included loot boxes. In December 2017 it was reported that Apple had recognised that gambling was being offered in this way and announced that any app in its App Store which offered loot boxes or the equivalent must disclose the odds of receiving any item prior to purchase. In June 2018 an editorial appeared in the academic journal *Addiction* warning of the dangers of loot boxes and other similar 'predatory monetisation schemes' (King & Delfabbro, 2018).

A second grey area is what the 2009 paper called non-monetary forms of gambling. For a start, it noted that many games included gambling situations and games of chance. Although these elements were usually optional, they were designed to 'entice the player to earn rewards quickly and further accelerate their progress in the game'. For example, in *Fable 2* the player was able to participate in a number of activities modelled on blackjack and roulette slot machines, and in *Grand Theft Auto: San Andreas*, players could enter a casino and play to win virtually unlimited amounts of in-game money.

An even more starkly obvious variety of non-monetary gambling is when traditional casino games like poker, blackjack and roulette are made available as stand-alone games which can be downloaded and played on a personal computer, mobile phone or dedicated game console using online services such as Microsoft's Xbox Live or by playing gambling apps on social networking sites such as Facebook. One of the most common non-monetary forms of gambling is when players can try out gambling games in the 'demo', 'practice' or 'free play' modes, with opportunities to do this on social networking sites four to five times more popular than those presented on real gambling sites (Ipsos Mori, 2009).

As King and colleagues (2009) pointed out, relevant regulators such as the Entertainment Software Rating Board in the USA and the Office of Film and Literature Classification in Australia, which aim to protect minors from material that is likely to harm or disturb them, are vigilant when it comes to anything that appears to condone or incite violence, particularly sexual violence, or which features alcohol or tobacco use, but generally overlook gambling or gambling-like content.

How a number of countries are struggling to control online gambling

Online gambling has faced governments with one of their greatest challenges in coming to terms with the digital world and its dangers. Table 1.2 shows examples of how a number of countries are struggling to control online gambling. This demonstrates how very differently countries have responded. The USA and Australia have opted for total or partial prohibition. But the USA in particular has felt the pressure to liberalise. In Germany, too, which has been the least permissive of all European countries when it comes to online gambling and where it has been illegal, there have also been moves to legalise the commercial online gambling industry.

TABLE 1.2 Examples of actions being taken by countries in an effort to control online gambling

Belgium[1]	A new regime, announced in 2018, would limit advertising of online gambling to operators' own websites or to existing customers; ban advertising during live sports broadcasts and within 15 minutes before or after any programmes aimed at minors; and ban use in adverts of athletes or celebrities with particular appeal for minors and advertisements via platforms or media targeted mainly at minors; also caps on the value of bonuses offered and amount accounts can be topped up per week
Sweden[2]	Gambling reform, coming into force in January 2019, will require the state monopoly to compete with the commercial sector for online gambling but will also bring in tighter regulation of gambling companies, collection of information about gambling behaviour and detection of risky patterns of gambling, the opportunity for players to set limits, a national self-exclusion register and a ban on advertising by unregistered companies
Switzerland[3]	A Money Gaming Act approved in 2017 will replace the country's existing gambling laws: it legalises online gambling, but only to be operated by locally licenced operators who have already established a land-based presence in the Swiss casino sector; foreign companies' websites will be blocked by Swiss internet service providers
Germany[4]	Online gambling remains illegal, and moves to legalise it require the agreement of all 16 individual states, the Länder, which have responsibility for gambling and vary in their approaches; there is a tradition of state ownership of lotteries, casinos and betting, and there is little call for privatisation despite lawsuits brought by companies against the Länder to the European Court of Justice
France[5]	Online lotteries are provided by a national monopoly only, and the online gambling regulator ARJEL grants licences only to providers with a physical address in France. They are only permitted to provide online sports betting, horse race betting and poker, considered less dangerous than pure chance games
Australia[6]	The 2018 Interactive Gambling Amendment Bill will ban all gambling advertisements during live sporting events broadcast between 5.00 am and 8.30 pm, beginning five minutes before start of play until five minutes after the end of the event, and will tighten the existing prohibition on providing any online gambling to Australian citizens apart from sports betting and lotteries – providing online poker, virtual machine gambling or bingo to Australians is illegal
USA[7]	Federal law bans online gambling, and the Unlawful Internet Gambling Enforcement Act (UIGEA) of 2006 brought in payment blocking, requiring credit card and other global payment systems to block payments to online gambling companies. In 2018, following a drawn-out legal challenge from the state of New Jersey, the Supreme Court was considering repealing the Professional and Amateur Sports Protection Act of 1992, which had largely outlawed sports betting

[1] CalvinAyre (2018a); [2] Cisneros Örnberg & Hettne (2018); [3] Yogonet Gaming News (2017b); [4] Loer (2018); [5] Marionneau & Berret (2018); [6] Hing *et al.* (2017), International Business Times (2018); [7] Sulkunen *et al.* (2019).

Historically, gambling regulation has taken very different routes in different European countries. The European Union ruling, after many legal challenges, is that, provided certain conditions are met, individual countries can regulate gambling in their own ways, including retaining the nationalisation of some or all gambling (see Chapter 2). While some European countries which have had government monopolies or monopoly concessions for operating at least a major part of their nations' gambling are moving in the direction of market liberalisation – Denmark is one such, where in 2017 Danske Spil's monopoly on offering online bingo and horse race betting was reportedly due to end (Yogonet Gaming News, 2017a) – other countries like Belgium have been moving to tighten their regulations.

Other Western European countries, such as Sweden and Switzerland, are also struggling with the question of how to manage the revolution in gambling, broadly speaking succumbing to the pressures to legalise commercial online gambling while at the same time trying to regulate gambling in such a way as to reduce the harm as far as possible. Many in those countries are rightly sceptical about whether these attempts at 'harm minimisation' are really tackling the underlying problem or are in effect covering up the continued growth of ever more danger-ous forms of gambling. For example, although consumer protection is claimed to be a cornerstone of the new Swedish system, where Svenska Spel's monopoly on online betting was ending, some are sceptical about its effectiveness in protecting against gambling harm for a number of reasons. For one thing the effectiveness of consumer protection, which they point out is couched in the language of 'respon-sible gambling' suggesting that the responsibility lies primarily with the gambler, depends very much on the way in which inspections, enforcement and penalties are implemented. There is also doubt about whether advertising controls will be effective in eliminating advertising by online companies registered in the UK and elsewhere (Cisneros Örnberg & Hettne, 2018). Opinions are also divided, I have been told, about whether the essentially liberalising new Swiss law does enough to protect citizens from gambling harm.

Resistance to the spread of casinos

In a number of countries, often beyond Europe, it has been the legalising of casinos that has figured large in the gambling debate. South Africa, Japan and Singapore are examples. A number of themes recur in these countries' stories.

One is the long-standing ambivalence that has characterised these countries' attitudes towards gambling, as indeed it has in almost all countries. For example, the Singapore Government and the ruling People's Action Party had deliberately put casinos at arm's length for many years. Indeed Singapore's late, revered leader Lee Kuan Yew once remarked that Singapore would have a casino 'over my dead body'. Despite surveys indicating that public opinion was divided, an online peti-tion with more than 30,000 signatures against the establishment of any casino in Singapore, and campaign group Families Against Casinos, the Government declined to hold a referendum and went ahead anyway (da Cunha, 2010).

Similarly in South Africa, the African National Congress (ANC) – traditionally critical of the homelands and of corrupt casinos – faced minimal public support for the liberalisation of gambling when it came to power. As we shall see, there is nothing unusual about citizens of a country mostly being opposed to gambling liberalisation – that turns out to be the case in all countries where serious efforts have been made to gauge public opinion. But public opinion appears to have played little role in the way South Africa's new liberalised gambling laws were formulated. In fact the argument was used that the right to gamble was a basic right denied citizens under apartheid and therefore consistent with black empowerment (Sallaz, 2009).

Another recurring theme is the unashamed prominence of governments' economic motives for legalisation. This was true for Singapore where, by the late 1990s, casinos were proposed as part of its new self-styled image as a 'Renaissance city of Asia'. The severe financial crisis the ANC faced was also undoubtedly a factor in South Africa when apartheid ended. The familiar justifications of promoting tourism and invigorating a floundering economy were again in evidence when the 2016 Japanese casino law was passed (Nippon.com, 2018). A related factor is the so-called domino effect. A factor in South Africa, as it so often has been in other places around the world, is that the country had closely neighbouring jurisdictions – the native 'homelands' to which white South Africans went to gamble – that had opted to legalise casino gambling. The spread of EGM gambling from New South Wales to Victoria in Australia, and casino gambling from one US state to another, are other examples. One's own citizens crossing a border to gamble looks to government treasuries like a loss of revenue that would be theirs if gambling opportunities could be brought home.

In China, Macau has been an exception to the prohibition of casino gambling since the first casino opened there in 1937 with the aim of attracting wealthy Chinese and European gamblers, later becoming officially a 'tourism and gaming region' (Schwartz, 2006). But Singapore's new casinos in the modern era have put domino-effect pressure on governments throughout its region. Vietnam is just one of a number of Asian countries that have liberalised their rules about casinos. Following the setting up of the casinos in Singapore, Vietnamese gamblers were going there to spend their money. Since this was money being lost to Vietnam, the new proposal was to reverse the policy which had tried to protect locals by making it illegal for them to play in Vietnamese casinos (World Casino News, 2018). Even India, which is a country where there has always been an ambivalent attitude towards gambling, has felt the influence of the setting up of casinos in Singapore and other Asian countries. Casinos, some 'floating' offshore, have opened in Goa; some other states, but not all, are following suit. Combined with the popularity of betting on sports such as cricket and state lotteries, gambling in India is now giving cause for concern (George *et al.*, 2014).

Another recurring theme has been governments' attempts to protect local citizens. A factor that persuaded Lew Kuan Yew to change his view and back the new casino resorts was the projection that two-thirds of revenue would be generated by tourists. Some attempt was made to protect locals from harm by the deterrent of having to pay a casino entrance fee. But, as Derek da Cunha pointed out in his 2010 book *Singapore Places Its Bets*, not all local residents would be deterred, and anyway hundreds of thousands of foreigners working in Singapore who were not permanent residents would be entitled to enter free of charge. The argument that large casinos are safe for local people because they largely cater for 'high-roller' outsiders has often been used to disarm opposition to the setting up of casinos. But the experience in many jurisdictions has been that long-term profitability is often dependent on those, sometimes insensitively referred to as the 'grind crowd', consisting of local low rollers. In South Africa, the recommendations of the early 1990s to protect the populace included that casinos should be placed an hour's drive from cities and limited to ten in number to insure against the 'over-stimulation of demand'. In Albania, a country with a particularly high prevalence of gambling problems (Molinaro *et al.*, 2014), Government decided to move casinos, as well as betting shops, out of residential areas altogether (AP News, 2018).

In 2017, the year after casinos were legalised in Japan, a number of articles appeared in the Japanese media criticising the Government's neglect of any countermeasures to combat gambling addiction which, according to one estimate, was affecting 700,000 Japanese each year and over three million at some point in their lives. Then, early in 2018, the *Japan Times* reported that the Government was considering a plan that would limit local residents to three casino visits per week and no more than 10 visits every 28 days. The rules would apply to Japanese nationals and foreigners living in Japan, while international tourists would be exempt. Local residents would be required to present identity cards to gain access to the casino floor (CalvinAyre, 2018b). These special rules for local are further good examples of how countries are struggling to reconcile the push for an international free market in gambling and the need to protect a nation's citizens from harm.

Pressure for gambling expansion is global and general

Almost all countries around the world are caught up in this, wavering between cashing in on what they see as a financial bonanza versus desperately trying to preserve their own cultural ways of doing things and to hold the line against the erosion of restraints on gambling which have existed in their countries to protect their citizens from harm. A good example of a country which finds itself in this dilemma is Brazil, which has a history of public interest in playing the popular Animal Game lottery and in horse racing but also one of widespread opposition to gambling and support for the prohibition of other forms of gambling. But it is no more immune than other countries to the pressure to legalise the now diverse range of new EGMs that exist in Brazil, the online gambling to which its citizens are exposed, plus a rapid expansion of electronic bingo. Legal battles over the future of gambling in Brazil are ongoing (Tavares, 2014).

Gambling is still officially prohibited in most Islamic countries, but this situation is changing rapidly. Casino gambling is allowed in Malaysia, for example, but only for tourists and non-Muslim locals (Sulkunen *et al.*, 2019). In North African countries, including Morocco, Algeria, Tunisia and Egypt, the question of whether gambling should continue to be outlawed is under active discussion as part of a wider debate about what kind of societies citizens want in the future (Toufiq, 2018).

I have concentrated in this chapter on EGM, online and casino gambling. But no aspect of gambling is unaffected by the rapid expansion of commercial gambling, the concern it has caused and the backlash it is giving rise to. Take as just one example, bingo – otherwise known in different countries over the years as loto, tombola, housey-housey and keno, and often thought of as 'not really gambling' or at least as a softer, more acceptable form of gambling, more popular with women. In some countries it has traditionally been associated more with charitable fundraising than with private profit. In several respects it is like lotteries (see Chapter 2 for a discussion of national lotteries) and in fact is treated as such under Irish law where it can only lawfully be offered by charitable and philanthropic organisations, unlike in Britain where the law also permits commercial organisations to offer bingo. But even bingo's reputation is not surviving unscathed. As Casey (2018) argues, the internet has challenged those perceptions of bingo as it has so much else about gambling. For one thing, the image of bingo as 'firmly rooted in national and local environments, and often associated with fun, neighbourliness, friendship, social interaction and community' has inevitably been diluted. Play itself has been transformed, being much faster and no longer involving marking of cards and 'calling' once a card is complete. Furthermore, as participants in Casey's research explained, charities had become dependent on private operators, often large international companies, to provide the technology necessary for them to offer online bingo, seen by some as thereby undermining their charitable ethos.

Signs that the era of unrestrained gambling liberalisation in Britain[1] may be coming to an end

Let us now turn to consider how the explosive growth of gambling and the resulting backlash has been working out in Britain.

An important event marking the beginning of the modern era of gambling liberalisation in Britain was the passing of the National Lottery Act in 1993. The restoration of a national lottery after over 150 years had needed to wait for the fall from power of Prime Minister Margaret Thatcher, who was virulently opposed to the state provision of gambling. But its restoration was sold on the idea that it did not really constitute gambling, since policy was still then governed by the philosophy that, while gambling had to be tolerated, it should not be positively encouraged. A key principle of Government regulation during this period was the so-called 'demand test'. Gambling promoters were allowed to meet existing demand but not to stimulate it. Proposals for new casinos and bingo clubs, for example, would be turned down unless they could provide evidence of existing unmet demand. Betting offices were not allowed to invite custom. The era of liberalisation, which Britain entered upon in the last years of the 20th century, consolidated by the 2005 Gambling Act, put paid to all that.

The last few years of the 20th century had witnessed a whole range of minor liberalising changes which did not require a change to primary legislation, but in 1999 the Labour Government set up a Gambling Review Body (GRB) which reported in 2001. The report, which made numerous recommendations for removing restrictions on gambling, was welcomed with delight by betting companies whose share prices rose instantly. Despite the complexity of the GRB report and the controversy surrounding many of its 176 recommendations, almost all of which were in the direction of liberalising the gambling laws, the large bulk of the recommendations was accepted by Government. Where recommendations were modified, they were nearly all modified in the direction of even greater derestriction than the GRB report recommended. The subsequent Act of 2005 set the overall regulatory framework for British gambling in the early 21st century.

Controversy has never been far away ever since. One issue which received a great deal of media attention at the time was the proposal, under the new Act, to open several mega-casino complexes. Extraordinary as it may seem now, the original Government proposal was for as many as 40 of these around the country, reduced under pressure to eight and finally to one. This was at first to be situated in Blackpool to help restore the fortunes of that iconic Victorian seaside town, and then in a poorer part of Manchester. Even that was finally stopped after a rebellion in Labour ranks and opposition from other parties, with Gordon Brown, shortly to take over as Prime Minister from Tony Blair, also against (Daily Mail, 2007).

The fob-tees maximum-stake debacle

After the casino resort idea was seen off, it was the presence in betting shops of Fixed Odds Betting Terminals (FOBTs), a form of gambling machine unknown until around the turn of the century, which was the feature of modern gambling which then made most of the news. After the inauguration of the national lottery, betting shops were claimed to be doing less well, and there was economic pressure to make moves to restore their position. Slot machines were allowed in betting shops for the first time in 1996, widely criticised by those who thought they were witnessing the death of the betting shop as they had known it.

But much worse was to come. The assumption had been that a customer could cope with about 40 betting events at most during a visit, but a new breed of entrepreneurs, with little or no interest in traditional horse or dog racing, saw the potential for greatly increased rapidity of betting. FOBTs had their origins in the provision of rapidly repeated lottery games controlled by a random number generator located remotely. It was successfully claimed that this rendered them legal:

the law forbade betting in a betting shop on any events taking place at the venue itself. But the betting companies saw the potential profits to be made from installing machines that allowed the playing of virtual forms of games, such as roulette and blackjack, to be found at casino tables. It was a tax change of 2001 which finally opened the way for the roulette machines: instead of the player being taxed, tax was now to be levied on the operator's profits (Hancock & Orford, 2014). Concerns were expressed, amongst the few who were aware of what was happening, that such machines might be even more addictive than slot machines. But this development, which has turned out to be so significant, never made the national news when the FOBTs were first introduced. It certainly did later.

Government and the betting companies struck a deal that allowed each betting shop to have up to four of the new type of machines. To the gambling regulator, the Gambling Commission (2019a), they are classed as B2 machines to distinguish them from other types of EGMs, but we have come to know them as the FOBTs or *fob-tees*. What was thought to be specially dangerous was the provision, since these were classed separately from other EGMs, for any amount to be staked up to a maximum of £100, unlike other EGMs where the maximum was £2. As we shall see, there is good reason to believe that the FOBTs are indeed every bit as dangerous as was thought. Mike Atherton, a journalist and former England test cricketer, wrote a highly informed book entitled simply, *Gambling*, in 2007, the year in which Britain's new liberalising Gambling Act came into operation. He referred specifically to how the FOBT machines had, 'changed the face of highstreet bookmaking. They have enabled the bookie to bypass laws that for years prevented them from hosting casino-style games'. He found the local bookmaker's shop to be utterly changed. One consequence was the starting of a campaign – The Fairer Gambling Campaign – which was very effective in getting the Government and other political parties to at least consider whether something should be done about them. The FOBT issue is the one that dominated debate about gambling policy in Britain during the few years leading up to the writing of this book. But it is just a reflection of what is going on the world over.

In 2017 an All Party Parliamentary Group (APPG) produced its report about the FOBTs. It heard evidence from people ranging from the Minister responsible for gambling at the Department for Culture, Media and Sport to those who had themselves experienced problems with the FOBTs. I was one of a number of academics who gave evidence. The bookmakers themselves were conspicuous by their absence, having declined to appear despite being given every opportunity to do so. The APPG concluded that there was 'widespread evidence of harm' associated with the FOBTs and that it was 'now time for the Government to act decisively to properly regulate FOBTs'. It should not wait for further research. Although it was not their only recommendation, the key one was that the maximum stake per go or 'spin' should be reduced to £2 on a precautionary basis until there was evidence that higher stakes were not harmful.

An example of increased media attention was *The Times* of 17 February 2016 which devoted part of its front page, a whole double-page inside spread and an editorial to gambling and specifically the FOBT machines, each of which it was calculated was making an annual profit of £48,000 – literally money-eating devices which extract £s from some people in order to put it in the pockets of others. There was by then widespread acknowledgement that something was wrong and needed to be changed. Sir Alan Budd, chair of the Review Body which preceded the 2005 Gambling Act, was on record as saying that having FOBTs in highstreet betting shops was not in the spirit of the Act. Even the Gambling Commission acknowledged that FOBTs constituted a 'hard' form of gambling. The APPG report was particularly critical of the Gambling Commission for having been slow off the mark in recognising the dangers of FOBTs. Other bodies, such as the influential and progressive British think tank the Institute for Public Policy Research (IPPR, 2016), joined in the accumulating calls for the FOBTs maximum-stake reduction.

Finally, in May 2018, after two consultations which had taken 18 months, Government bowed to the concerted pressure for change and announced its intention to cap the FOBT stake size at £2. That was not the end of the matter, however, since the Treasury anticipated loss of revenue; putting the change into effect was to be delayed by a further two years. In the Government's budget statement of October 2018, the implementation date was brought forward to October 2019, still a whole year's further delay after years of inaction in the face of mounting evidence and pressure. The junior minister responsible for sport and gambling, who it was known had faced an uphill struggle to get the change implemented, could put up with it no longer and resigned in early November 2018. In her letter of resignation to the Prime Minister, she ominously told the PM the delay was 'due to commitments made by others to those with registered interests' (The Guardian, 2018b). We shall see in later chapters how industry and its allies resist reforms, of which the FOBT stake reform is such a notable example, by trying to get us to think about gambling in a way that is least challenging to their interests (Chapter 3) and by attempting to control research on the subject and how research results are interpreted (Chapter 8).

Although it was the *fob-tees* that had the lion's share of media attention, concern was building up which extended well beyond that one form of gambling device. In their important 2016 report, the IPPR estimated that gambling problems were costing Government up to a billion pounds a year in excess healthcare, crime and benefits costs and loss of tax income alone, not to mention the more personal and less tangible costs (see chapters 6 and 7). They concluded by calling for a national Government strategy to tackle problem gambling and reduce gambling-related harm which, they said, should be seen as a public health issue.

In September 2018, after their own consultation, a number of such suggestions were taken up by the Labour Party opposition, which announced some of the things it would do if it came into Government. One was the all-important suggestion that Britain now needed a new Gambling Act. Nothing illustrates better the controversy which continues to surround gambling and the backlash which the lifting of previous restraints on gambling inevitably provokes. Little more than ten years after a liberalising Act came into operation, one of the country's main political parties was calling for a new one. Nor is the taste for change limited to one political party. This speaks volumes about the mistakes that were made – under a Labour administration, ironically – when unthinkingly and so comprehensively liberalising gambling around the turn of the century. The era of thoughtless derestriction of gambling may be coming to an end sooner than one might have thought.

There were even signs that the *Gambling Establishment* was getting the message. The CEO of the Gambling Commission (2017), in her annual conference address to the industry, had this to say:

> The last 12 months . . . have witnessed increased interest in gambling from politicians, the press and most importantly, from the public . . . we have seen an intensification of the debate and concerns around the costs of gambling – the hidden addiction; the ubiquity of gambling, in particular around children and young people; and the fitness of this sector to respond to shifting public opinion. . . . Looking honestly at your businesses, with open minds, have you done enough? I think the need is more pronounced now than it has ever been, and the bald facts are that you haven't done enough to demonstrate to us that you're there yet. . . . In excess of two million people in Britain are at risk or classed as problem gamblers . . . we are not seeing those numbers come down. . . . Gambling related harm is a public health issue. . . . The true cost for some people and their families is devastating.

The Commission started to mete out some hefty fines. For example, William Hill was fined over £6m and the online betting firm 32Red over £1m for 'money laundering and social responsibility failures' – in other words not properly checking how players who had deposited over half a million pounds over a period of several months could be financing their betting from their moderate incomes (Gambling Commission, 2018a, 2018b). In the William Hill case, several players turned out to be criminals using betting to launder money. In the 32Red case, the Commission reported that the person concerned had displayed numerous signs of having a serious gambling problem which had not been picked up.

Intensification of the long-held concern in Britain about gambling and young people

Concern about its effect on the young has always been close to the centre of the debate about gambling. In his thorough and excellent book about the history of British commercial gambling regulation, law professor David Miers (2004) has much to say about this. He reminds us that anti-gambling groups, active in the first half of the 20th century, argued all along that gambling had a morally debilitating effect on the young. The moral argument was less often heard in later years, but between the 1960s and late 1980s, in the era of tolerance-without-encouragement of gambling, concern about young people came up again. In Britain, the worry now was about young people playing gambling machines in 'amusement arcades' which operated unclear and inconsistent age controls. They were attractive places for young people in those days. A report by the National Housing and Town Planning Council in 1988, for example, found that over half of its sample of 10,000 children visited amusement arcades.

The issue of children's access to gambling machines was still a live one at the very end of the century when the Government was seeking support for its policy of liberalising gambling regulation. In fact it was the single issue on which opinion was most divided amongst members of the Gambling Review Body which advised the Government at the time. There still existed a peculiarly British anomaly of allowing children of any age to play low-stake/low-prize EGMs. The Committee thought hard about this issue but in the end recommended that the anomalous conditions should remain, as they do to this day. EGMs would be categorised according to stake and prize sizes. The ones that children could play, euphemistically termed 'amusement with prizes' or AWP machines, would be 'category D'. According to Miers (p 508):

> Many believed that the government was sending out an unclear message by allowing children to gamble on the lower value AWP machines, while simultaneously claiming that gaming machines and children should not mix. The new categories of gaming machines would, it was argued, confuse parents, children, and the machine operators themselves.

Miers was critical of the Department for Culture, Media and Sport which, in the absence of firm evidence that children were being harmed, did not feel that removing them was justified. He thought the distinction that the Government was making between category D machines that they thought were safe for children, and other types of EGMs which were not, was 'artificial and disingenuous'. He thought category D machines were likely to be effective as 'devices for acquiring the gambling habit' and would be a danger to children.

Access for children remained an issue for other forms of gambling as well. For example, there were no restrictions on children's access to members' clubs, which were allowed to have jackpot machines (known in Britain's arcane regulatory system as category B4 machines). Under 18s can also be present on bingo premises, provided that they don't take part in the game. But that doesn't make it unlawful for them to play on the machines that are sited there. There is no age limit on a child's access to a pub or an amusement arcade in a city centre or motorway service area, where control is much more difficult and likely to vary from place to place. Where premises are allowed machines in both category D and category C (adult-only machines with larger stakes and prizes), separation of the areas housing the different types of machine is problematic.

Those are particular British issues, but the bigger concern that is building about the risks of gambling to British children and young people are those that were discussed in a global context earlier in this chapter – the phenomenal growth of online gambling, its widening links with popular sports, the grey area between social media and gambling, and the general normalisation of gambling.

Citizens find their voice

British citizens are starting to make their views heard on the subject. Some of those who have posted comments on my Gambling Watch UK website[2] have told heartrending personal stories of their own descent into debt and depression through gambling (gambling addiction is the subject of Chapter 6). Others have told of their agonising worry about someone else in the family (covered in Chapter 7). Suicidal thoughts and intentions, and stories of the actual suicides of gambling relatives and friends, constitutes a common theme. Some express great sadness. Others are angry. But one of the largest categories of comments have consisted of criticisms of gambling policy, critical of the Government and parts of the gambling industry. A common theme is what is seen as Government 'greed', its gambling tax gains, its 'shame' in allowing the present situation, mistakes by previous Governments, the danger of an 'epidemic' of gambling problems and the dangers for 'future generations'. The following are typical:

> I think that there should be a serious attempt to lobby Government to change the laws on gambling advertisements of all kinds. Gambling addiction is a life threatening disease. There is such a deep focus on keeping cigarettes out of people's hands and constantly showing adds about what nicotine does to your body followed by ones that tell you to HURRY and place online bets!! I don't see why gambling is not focused on as much. . . . I hope campaigners look into this matter more seriously and try and implement stricter regulations around it.
>
> The prevalence of the bookmakers on our streets in the UK is the toxic result of weak decision making by our politicians. What happened to us here in the UK!? I wonder if other countries' leaders have allowed their population to also be exposed and vulnerable to this type of exploitation. The Labour government made a massive error and breached their duty of care for many people by allowing the gambling industry to open a new assault on their target customers through FOBTs, and the current administration has done nothing to try and repair the damage to my knowledge.

Gambling with Lives (GwL)[3] is a group started by the parents of a young man with a gambling addiction who committed suicide. They are naturally grief stricken but also very angry at the way they believe their son was, in their words, groomed and targeted by the online gambling industry, and at the Government which is doing so little about this. An extensive piece based around an interview they gave appeared in the national British press in June 2018 (Daily Mail, 2018a). They have been joined by others who have experienced the same kind of tragic bereavements through gambling, and GwL was officially launched at Westminster in November 2018. GwL's stated priorities include raising awareness of the potentially fatal consequences of gambling; £2 to be the maximum stake for *all* online slot and casino betting; gambling to be seen as a public health issue; the levy on the gambling industry for prevention, treatment and research to be greatly increased to 1% of gross profits; and NHS treatment to be hugely increased and to include support for families. There is substantial overlap between those suggestions and my own manifesto for gambling reform set out in Chapter 9.

Dissatisfaction with British gambling policy is by no means confined to those who have experienced the most acute gambling-related tragedies. Citizens in general tend to be conscious of actual or potential harms from gambling. Even while the UK Government was busy preparing for its major 2005 liberalising gambling legislation, a 2003 survey carried out by National Opinion Poll suggested that British public opinion was not in favour of further liberalisation. For example, 93% said 'Yes' to the question *Do you think there are enough opportunities for people to gamble in Britain at the moment?* The 2007 British Gambling Prevalence Survey included questions about attitudes towards gambling (Wardle *et al.*, 2007). The results were clear-cut. Although most people were not in favour of prohibition of gambling, the weight of public opinion was on the side of believing that gambling is dangerous; that on balance it is bad rather than good for families, communities and society as a whole; and that it should not be encouraged. For example, 65% agreed that 'Gambling is dangerous for family life' (only 8% disagreed), and 55% disagreed that 'On balance gambling is good for society' (only 8% agreed). Although there were differences in attitudes between different groups of citizens – for example men were more positive towards gambling than women, younger people were more positive than older, and frequent gamblers more positive than others – all socio-demographic groups, and even gamblers as a group, were on balance negative in their attitudes (Orford *et al.*, 2009). Australia, Canada, Israel and Finland are other countries where public attitudes towards gambling have been assessed with similar results (Australian Productivity Commission, 1999; Azmier, 2000; Gavriel-Fried, 2015; Salonen *et al.*, 2014).

The 2010 British Gambling Prevalence Survey repeated the exercise and found that, although attitudes towards gambling had changed very slightly in a more positive direction, the general picture was the same (Wardle *et al.*, 2011). Survey data collected by the Gambling Commission since then, using the same set of questions, has shown that attitudes towards gambling have been getting even slightly more negative. At the same time, the proportion of people who think that 'in this country gambling is conducted fairly and can be trusted' declined steadily each year between 2012 and 2018 from just under 50% to only 30% (Gambling Commission, 2019a).

The backlash is under way

In Britain and around the world voices are being raised expressing alarm at how commercially provided gambling has been allowed to grow and flourish in the few decades at the end of the 20th and beginning of the 21st centuries. Countries have been struggling to cope with the emergence of more technologically sophisticated gambling machines spreading into bars, clubs and highstreets; the exposure of their citizens to numerous companies advertising online gambling; or the spectre of casino gambling in places where such a thing is not traditional. National, regional and local governments have been faced with dilemmas about what to do. Committees, think tanks and the media have addressed the issues. Grass roots campaign groups have formed and made noise. The general public, when asked, is negative about the growth of gambling. All are worried about the possibility of increasing addiction to gambling, the intrusiveness of gambling advertising and the way gambling seems to be becoming normal. The thing that all express greatest concern about is the effect on a country's children and young people.

We have seen in this chapter that there is now evidence of a growing backlash against the continued expansion of gambling. Some countries have been finding ways to reduce the numbers or dangerousness of gambling machines or ways to limit the exposure to their citizens to online gambling or casinos. In Britain, which from 2005 became one of Europe's most liberal gambling regimes, there are signs that the tide is turning. The backlash is under way. However, the power of what I shall call the *Gambling Establishment* – the gambling industry and its allies inside and outside Government – is formidable, and it will certainly fight back. In the next two chapters we will look in more detail at this powerful alliance: in Chapter 2 at some of the details of its size and structure; in Chapter 3 at its ideology, its favoured beliefs which it has tried to disseminate amongst us.

Notes

1 The Gambling Commission regulates commercial gambling in Great Britain (England, Scotland and Wales). Gambling is regulated separately in Northern Ireland.
2 www.gamblingwatchuk.org
3 www.gamblingwithlives.com

2

THE GAMBLING ESTABLISHMENT

The industry and its allies inside and outside government

In Chapter 1 we saw how commercial gambling, always controversial, became much more so in the first years of the 21st century, to the point at which it is now provoking the backlash which some predicted. In this chapter I want to take a look at where the push for more and more gambling and more dangerous gambling is coming from. Obviously that is from the profit-making industry. But governments that have supported an expansionist industry are also heavily implicated, as, too, are a range of non-government organisations which knowingly or inadvertently support them. I use the expression the *Gambling Establishment* to refer to this powerful alliance of interests which collectively has been responsible for the modern growth in gambling and therefore for the harm it is causing. Let us begin with the industry.

The gambling industry

The size of the world gambling market

Commercial gambling is now on a colossal scale. The size of the global gambling industry in 2016 and 2017 in terms of gross gambling revenue (GGR: the sum of all money gambled minus the winnings returned to players) was just short of US$400 billion annually (The Economist, 2017; The New York Times, 2018; Sulkunen *et al.*, 2019). The country that contributed the most to that total was the USA (about $115 billion), followed in order by China (including Macau and Hong Kong), Japan, Italy, Australia and then Britain with a total GGR of $18 billion.[1] Probably more important, however, is how those figures work out per adult in the different countries. When that is calculated, two countries easily outstrip all others, Australia and Singapore, with an amount lost to gambling per capita annually in the region of $1,000. Third place went to Ireland at about

$500 and then Finland, the USA, New Zealand, each at $400–500, followed by Canada, Norway, Italy and Britain, each at $300–400 per person. In gambling business terms this is revenue, but to individuals who gamble these are losses. Bearing in mind that many people gamble very little or not at all and that the way losses are distributed across a country's population is very skewed – something that we shall want to look at more closely in Chapter 5 – these figures suggest that there are many people who are contributing large amounts of money to gambling industry profits.

Market growth in the first years of the century was greatest in the Asia-Pacific and North American regions of the world, with only modest growth in Africa and Latin America. Among changes in the five years from 2013 were steady increases in GGR in Australia, Britain and Ireland; steady increases in Norway after a substantial fall associated with reform of electronic gambling machines (EGMs) between 2005 and 2009; a fairly stable picture in the USA, Canada and New Zealand; and some fall in GGR in Italy after a dramatic increase between 2003 and 2011.

Those figures mask sizeable differences in the form that commercial gambling takes in different countries. The Australian market is dominated by gambling machines, the 'pokies', situated outside casinos, as it is in Italy and New Zealand also. Casinos dominate in Singapore and the USA and to a lesser extent in Canada and Malta and are a big sector in Australia and New Zealand. Lotteries are a substantial sector in many countries and one of the biggest sectors in Cyprus, Iceland, Malta, Sweden and Italy. Online gambling is one of the sectors that has grown most in the previous ten years. It has become the largest sector in Ireland, Britain and each of the Scandinavian countries. Betting is a significant component in many countries, although it is much larger in some, such as Ireland and Australia. The UK has a particularly diverse gambling market, outstripping other European countries for betting and bingo but also having amongst the largest casino, lottery and gambling-machine industries (Eadington, 2008).

The online gambling contribution

By the start of the second decade of the new century the estimated economic value of the online gambling industry was over US$20 billion, with online poker being the fastest growing sector, estimated at over $6 billion. In Italy alone, the total market for legal online gambling, in GGR, was €9.4 billion by 2015, with a large illegal market estimated at €1.3 billion. In the UK, licenced online gambling generated a GGR of £4.5 billion in 2016–2017. Restrictions on sports and online betting in the USA had left the international market clear for domination by large UK and Irish-based companies such as bet365 and Paddy Power Betfair, the latter the result of a £5 billion merger of Paddy Power and Betfair in 2016. Another among a spate of company mergers in the 2010s was the £1.1 billion acquisition in 2015 of Bwin.party by GVC, the owners of Sportingbet. William Hill and Paddy Power were the two largest online gambling companies in 2015, valued at US$5.2 billion and 3.8 billion respectively. Seven other companies had market capitalisations over $1 billion (Financial Times, 2017; The Guardian, 2017; Sulkunen *et al.*, 2019). This is truly big business.

Company mergers and acquisitions and increased concentration have been trends in the gambling industry generally. In the USA, the industry is heavily concentrated in a small number of large operators located in Las Vegas or on the East Coast. Most of the world's 12 largest, highly profitable casino companies, such as Las Vegas Sands, MGM Resorts and Caesar's Entertainment, are based in the USA. UK-based companies, often operating through low-tax jurisdictions outside the European Union, are major players in both land-based and online forms of gambling. Sulkunen *et al.* (2019), drawing on a report for the European Union, tell us that UK bookmakers William Hill and Ladbrokes each have clients in over 150 countries. Ladbrokes, for example, offers online gambling services in 11 languages. In 2017–18 the acquisition of Ladbrokes Coral by GVC and of Sky Betting & Gaming by the Stars Group contributed to the industry's consolidation. By 2016, three big companies accounted for no less than 87% of the British sports betting retail market, and five accounted for 84% of the online betting market (Lopez-Gonzalez *et al.*, 2018a). Austria is another country where gambling companies are big players internationally (Bereiter & Storr, 2018). Casinos Austria controls Casinos Austria International, which operates casinos in 14 countries, including in Egypt and Palestinian territories, and on six US cruise liners as well as in European countries. One of the largest private companies, the Austrian Novomatic Group, is one of the world's biggest gambling companies, operating over 2,000 online casino and betting establishments worldwide. The leading pan-European sportsbook is an Austrian-based bookmaker, Win2Day, operating out of Gibraltar under UK jurisdiction. Sizable rivals include Sportingbet, UK-based but operating from Antigua, and such others as Betfred (UK), Punt Club (Australia, a social betting service), Openbet (UK), Unibet, and 888 holdings (Gibraltar) (Sulkunen *et al.*, 2019).

Some individuals have become very wealthy in the process. They include James Packer and Len Ainsworth, reportedly among the richest men in Australia, who acquired their wealth through the profits of casinos and online operator Crown-Bet (which made Au$490 million profit in 2013), and Aristocrat Leisure, which manufactures slot machines and other gambling technology (Markham & Young, 2014b; Sulkunen *et al.*, 2019). Denise Coates owns online gambling company bet365. Her 2017–18 annual income of £265 million was widely reported in the British media as being the highest figure for remuneration of a head of any UK company of any kind (Independent, 2018). An article in *The Times* in February 2016 produced a revelation about the wealth the gambling business has generated for the family (uncles, brother) of the UK's then Chancellor of the Exchequer, George Osborne.

Industry and its aspirations

Although much of gambling companies' plans remains hidden behind a wall protective of trade secrets, the industry is quite open about its expansionist aspirations in general. Since it is treated by governments and regulators as a bone fide industry, and therefore one to be encouraged, this is not surprising. I gained some insight into the ambitions of the UK online gambling industry when a few years ago I attended an industry seminar on the subject – not the kind of occasion that, as an academic, I had been used to attending (Westminster eForum, 2012). It was an opportunity for me to eavesdrop on their discussions and to ask one or two questions myself. I came away with further clues about how the industry thinks, the language it talks and how it is going about making the case for further expansion of online gambling. A recurrent theme was the repeated call for 'harmonisation' of online gambling regulation across Europe. This came from the Secretary General of the European Gaming and Betting Association and from several other speakers. Countries such as France, Germany and Belgium were depicted as 'resistant' and 'protectionist', possibly flouting EU law. Britain, in contrast, was repeatedly cited as being the leader in online gambling in Europe, where the industry was 'fiercely competitive, successful, well-established', a model for the rest of the continent. Concern was expressed that the UK might back down from its position as 'the arch free marketeer', bringing in 'over-regulation' and a level of taxation which might throttle innovation and stifle growth of the industry.

The British online gambling industry has been given every reason to think that its innovation and expansion is welcome and encouraged. Its assertive stance towards Europe is therefore only to be expected. It is nevertheless very concerning. There was no acknowledgement that the different regimes in different European countries were partly a consequence of differences in cultures and traditions and reflected valid concerns about the need to protect citizens from the likely harmful consequences of exposing them to new forms of gambling. There was repeated reference to 'consumer protection', but this was never defined, and it appeared to refer more to consumers being well-informed about products and being given a choice of fair and attractive products rather than to an awareness of the inherently dangerous nature of the products themselves.

I have also become used to reading in some detail UK Government reports on the subject – again, not something that would have been high-priority reading for me earlier in my career. One very telling document was produced by the Government Department for Digital, Culture, Media and Sport (DCMS, 2017b) summarising evidence it had received in response to its first consultation document of 2016 on the subject of, among other things, possible changes to EGMs, including the by then notorious FOBTs (Fixed Odds Betting Terminals or category B2 EGMs: see Chapter 1). I wasn't surprised to read that industry responses had been against reducing the maximum FOBT stake from £100 to £2, since everyone accepted that this would inevitably reduce the profits from these now most highly profitable EGMs. What intrigued me, though, were the *increases* in stakes and availability of gambling which the industry was suggesting elsewhere. While attention was focussed on the *fob-tees*, it was being proposed that expansion be pursued elsewhere while media and others' attention was diverted. For example, the industry proposed increases in maximum stakes on other categories of

EGM (B3, C and D category machines) and also proposed a 400% increase (from £20,000 to £100,000) in the maximum progressive jackpot prize for B1 machines in casinos (as well as proposing that jackpots should be allowed to be accumulated across casinos for the first time) and increases in prizes in categories C and D.

The iconic British pub is another ubiquitous gambling venue. Many pubs, but by no means all, take up their allowance of having two category C machines. The British Beer and Pub Association, supported by BACTA (the British Amusement Catering Trades Association), proposed increases in maximum stake on these machines from £1 to £2 and maximum prize from £100 to £250. Accountancy firm PricewaterhouseCoopers (PwC) estimated this would contribute to the often waning economic viability of British pubs by generating £72 million, as well as £10 million in tax revenue and benefit to machine manufacturers (DCMS, 2017a).

BACTA also argued that category C machines in gambling arcades – officially termed 'adult entertainment centres' – were not economically viable. They then made a further extraordinary suggestion which indicates the way they were thinking. They proposed a new sub-category of machine for the arcades, a B5, which would have a maximum stake of £10, a maximum prize of £125, and a spin cycle of 30 seconds. This, they argued, would allow operators to offer a more varied selection of products including what they described as 'low stake roulette'. In support of this proposal, PwC estimated that the manufacture of 10,000 such machines would generate economic benefit of £165 million and increased taxes of £25 million (DCMS, 2017a). So, while facing criticism and likely tighter regulation over the FOBTs, which had effectively brought casino-type gambling on to British highstreets, turning betting shops into mini casinos, sections of the industry were busy plotting to do the same with Britain's other highstreet gambling venue, the amusement arcade!

Regarding category D machines, the so-called 'amusements with prizes' which Britain, unlike other jurisdictions, allows children to play, PwC showed their colours by claiming that evidence of harm to young people from playing such machines is inconclusive. It is interesting to note that the whole of the relevant chapter of the report was written from the point of view of 'markets' and with reliance on PwC for the estimate of financial effects of changes. To their credit, DCMS was not persuaded about the need for these changes 'at this time'. Amongst their reasons were: B3s are now the fastest growing gambling machines sector and player protection is important; pubs constitute a 'less regulated environment' and are 'ambient' gambling establishments; and, when it comes to category D, there continues to be concern about the possible link between gambling early in life and later gambling problems.

In September 2018, a seminar was held in London entitled 'Next Steps for the UK Gambling Industry – Innovation, Regulation and the Future Shape of the Sector'. Several speakers at the meeting were asking how the industry was going to respond to the backlash against unrestrained commercial gambling and the prospect of greater regulation. As one delegate is reported to have said:

The UK gambling sector, particularly the iGaming sector, is often portrayed as a stand out industry globally in terms of innovation and talent, creating some of the world's leading brands, products, and services. But as we look to export this innovation and capability to new markets, how will we ensure the UK industry can continue to grow in the next decade with these significant regulatory headwinds?

(Westminster eForum, 2018, p 31)[2]

On the specific issue of the threat to the industry from the recent Government decision to prohibit high stakes on FOBT machines, the industry anticipated inevitable betting shop closures and job losses. But one view was that the industry would not want to part with such large and valuable retail estates. This was an opportunity to change and diversify. If local authorities thought that the new FOBT legislation would rid the highstreet of a lot of its betting offices – something a large number of local councils have been arguing for – then they were going to be disappointed, it was said. In fact it appears they might see yet more gambling venues on their highstreets: Ladbrokes Coral had already opened some 'adult gaming centres', and other major companies were thought to be contemplating the same. The idea that the threat of greater regulation could be met by diversifying was a general theme of the meeting. As another delegate put it:

You've then got new opportunities, you've got new products coming on line, you've got new markets, you've got new regulation, and that gives you a chance to diversify . . . so let's diversify our business model, make it more flexible, make it less rigid, less exposed to risk.

(Westminster eForum, 2018, p 24[2])

The UK online gambling industry was also very focussed on the repeal of the legislation in the USA which would pave the way for individual states to legalise sports betting. There were predictions of a US market estimated as worth up to $6 billion in annual gross gambling revenues. The meeting was cautious, however. Sports betting, it was pointed out, was still only available in a minority of states, and US state regulation had tended to reinforce the position of existing land-based operators such as casinos and racetracks. With the exception of Paddy Power's acquisition of FanDuel, European operators had been cautious about moving in to the US market and had focussed on strategic partnerships such as William Hill with Eldorado and GVC with MGM.

The industry continued to complain about how countries across the European Union were still permitted to pursue their own ways of dealing with gambling. One country referred to with approval was Sweden, moving towards a commercial market opening early in 2019, modelled in part on British and Danish regimes and already open for online gambling licence applications. Meanwhile Germany and the Netherlands, also significant potential markets, remained from the industry perspective unreformed, hinting at the possible introduction of an online licencing regime but not acting decisively, leaving things at best confusing for the industry.

Governments

Governments, often working with the commercial sector, as gambling providers

The ways in which governments get involved in gambling are complex, diverse, changeable and often mysterious to the general public and even to those who take a special interest in the subject. One rather paradoxical fact is that many governments, which have a primary duty to protect their citizens, actually provide gambling themselves. In fact, a number of countries have had at least partial state or state-supported gambling monopolies which continue to exist in some European and other countries, although sometimes in modified form. Finland is one such country. Veikkaus continues to have a monopoly on the lottery and betting business other than horse race betting, which is operated by a separate state-regulated company, and RAY, Finland's Slot Machine Association, has a monopoly on EGMs and casino games including online casino game playing. No other company has the legal right to operate gambling in Finland. Foreign competition is banned, the exception being a slot machine association which has a right to offer various forms of gambling on Åland, an autonomous part of Finland, and on board ships (Tammi *et al.*, 2015). Other Scandinavian countries, Canada, the Netherlands, Luxembourg, Switzerland, Slovakia and Hong Kong are further examples of countries with strong traditions of having government gambling monopolies. But it is nearly always the case that the monopoly covers only certain types of gambling, sitting alongside other forms of gambling that are operated legally by commercial companies or charities or which are being offered illegally (Sulkunen *et al.*, 2019).

State lotteries are the most often protected national gambling monopolies and important public-revenue generators even in countries with otherwise competitive gambling markets. A cross-national comparative study of 125 state lotteries found that 48% of jurisdictions had licenced a private company to operate a monopoly lottery. Another 48% had state-owned companies or ran lotteries directly through a designated ministry or department. In some cases national lotteries are licenced to non-profit organisations. The majority of countries in Africa, Asia and South America had contracted their national lotteries to private operators, whereas in Europe and North America the majority of jurisdictions had government-operated lotteries (Gidluck, 2016).

The National Lottery in the UK is a good example of a lottery run on behalf of a government by a private company. This arrangement whereby a government grants permission to a single commercial or other non-state organisation to provide a particular form of gambling – the Australian state of Victoria granting a single licence for a casino is another example – has obvious attractions for governments.

It creates a monopoly with no price competition, allows greater profit surplus and produces generous government revenue which can be allocated to 'good causes' such as the development of culture and sport or even for such things as scientific research, education, and health and social care provided by non-government charities. It has been said that this has provided a convenient 'alibi' for governments legalising gambling more generally (Lepper & Creigh-Tyte, 2013; Kingma, 2004).

The complexity of the interplay between governments and commerce in the operation of gambling is compounded in countries which divide responsibility between national and regional or provincial governments. Austria is a country which illustrates as well as any the complexity of gambling regulation and the tortuous arguments about the nature of gambling that are so often involved (Bereiter & Storr, 2018). It has a federal state monopoly on 'games of chance', including games in casinos and the national lottery, operated, respectively, by Casinos Austria and Österreichische Lotterien. Forms of gambling depending more on skill such as sports betting are regulated by the nine Austrian provinces. Needless to say, the distinction is by no means clear-cut. For example, a combination sports bet, depending on the outcome of several events combined, is ruled to be largely a matter of chance and comes under the state monopoly system, whereas a single bet is considered to involve a large measure of skill and comes within the provinces' purview. How EGMs are dealt with is equally peculiar. The monopoly covers EGMs in casinos as well as all Video Lottery Terminals, which to appearances are much like other EGMs but which, like the British FOBTs, are 'terminals' in the sense that outcomes are determined remotely. Other EGMs, where outcomes are determined within the machine itself, are regulated by the provinces, although only five have established a system for licencing EGM providers, whereas the other four provinces, including Vienna, prohibit them.

Illegal gambling

Those who argue for 'channelling' gambling towards a regulated and taxed activity can point to the size of illegal gambling markets. In their international review, Sulkunen et al. (2019) provide a number of examples. One estimate, for example, was that in 2014 80% of the global sports betting market was illegal. In the USA, for example, since few states, until very recently, allowed sports betting, it was estimated in 2017 that US citizens wagered approximately $150 billion on illegal online gambling sites. In Germany, the Government estimated in 2012 that the annual turnover of the unauthorised sports betting market was €2.7 billion, 60% of it online betting. Slovakia is another example of an EU country where the large majority of online players were thought to be mostly gambling on unauthorised foreign sites. Other examples of unauthorised gambling include illegal EGMs, as well as computer terminals that have been turned into gambling machines, common in bars in southern France, Greece and Spain, and mafia-controlled gambling machines in Italian pubs. The illegal Brazilian animal lottery, *Jogo do Bicho*, has been estimated to collect almost 60% more revenue than legal lotteries. In India, clandestine lottery sales account for about half the Indian gambling market of an estimated annual US$60 billion.

Regulation, EU and WTO rules

By its very nature, unregulated, usually cross-border, online gambling, dramatically increased in volume, has posed a particular dilemma for governments. Most countries in Western Europe have moved to legalising and licencing online gambling, even where there had been long-established monopoly systems. Norway, for example, legalised some form of online gambling in 2004, the UK in 2005, France and Italy in 2010, Spain in 2011, Denmark in 2012 and Portugal in 2015. But countries have differed in how they have dealt with providers based outside their own jurisdictions. Some have opted for 'closed regulation', restricting licencing to domestic gambling providers, while others have chosen 'open regulation', also allowing operators based elsewhere to market online gambling to their citizens. France is an example of relatively closed regulation. Online lotteries are provided by a national monopoly only, and the online gambling regulator ARJEL grants licences only to providers with a physical address in France. They are only permitted to provide online sports betting, horse race betting and poker, considered less dangerous than pure chance games. The UK, by contrast, is an example of open regulation, although it was deemed necessary to follow the 2005 Gambling Act, which opened up the market to domestic and offshore providers, with the Gambling (Licensing and Advertising) Act in 2014. Operators are required to be licenced and monitored by the regulator, the Gambling Commission, and can accept wagers from the UK and anywhere else in the world but are now subject to a 'point-of-consumption' tax of 15% whenever gambling revenue originates in the UK (Gambling Act, 2014). Portugal's new system is a hybrid: to be licenced, online gambling operators would be required to have at least a subsidiary company based in Portugal.

There have been regular indications of how contested has become the issue of whether regulations should be harmonised across the countries of the European Union (Sulkunen et al., 2019; Verbiest, 2007). For example, the European Court of Justice had upheld the right of German states to block an online gambling company from providing its services to German citizens. But at the same time it had ruled that Italy was acting in contradiction to EU free-trade rules by prohibiting or restricting cross-border online gambling. Austria also provides a good example of a country that has struggled with the issue of meeting EU rules. The latter support individual countries pursuing their own national regimes, provided controls are proportionate and justified in terms of ensuring consumer protection, not just on grounds of protecting the home country's own industry and source of revenue income (Bereiter & Storr, 2018). Whether Austria's partial gambling monopoly fulfilled the EU requirements was considered in 2016 by each of its three highest courts – Administrative, Constitutional, and Supreme Court on Civil and

Criminal Matters – which, after a lengthy process, concluded that the monopoly *was* compatible with EU law.

Similar disputes had taken place in the USA, which for some time stood out against the legalisation of online gambling. But following a Justice Department ruling that existing gambling law only covered sports betting, Nevada, New Jersey and Delaware legalised intrastate online gambling in 2013, and by 2015 several other states were considering following suit. But the issue provoked a backlash focussed on worries about crime and money laundering and potential harmful effects on youngsters and problem gamblers, and a bill to restore a ban on online gaming was introduced in Congress seeking to reinstate federal law to prohibit all forms of internet gambling. In one state, New Jersey, where one prediction was that the state's online gambling market could be generating over $400 million by 2017 (Online Casino City, 2015), online gambling sites stopped accepting their own residents as customers after being warned. The World Trade Organisation, whose rule is that a nation limiting foreign supply of gambling services can only be justified on grounds of protecting morality, public order, health and human life, and essential security interests, judged illegal the USA's prohibition of offshore-provided online gambling. The USA has chosen to ignore their decision. Meanwhile, Sulkunen *et al.*'s (2019) opinion is that the USA has been relatively successful in prohibiting online gambling, using the Unlawful Internet Gambling Enforcement Act (UIGEA) of 2006 which brought in payment blocking, requiring credit card and other global payment systems to block payments to online gambling companies.

Governments' dependence on gambling

There are strong economic incentives for governments to legalise and licence gambling, including online gambling. However it is collected, whether as a business tax, licencing fees, a tax on gross gambling revenue (GGR), a tax on admission to gambling venues (as is often the case in the USA), a tax on players' winnings (as in the UK before 2001) or in some other way, government treasuries have a huge stake in the promotion and growth of gambling. In the process, governments can become heavily dependent on gambling income. One estimate is that gambling produces a public revenue of €85 billion in the EU, and the position is similar in several other parts of the world. Many countries, including Canada and Australia, collect amounts of revenue from gambling that now rival those collected from alcohol and tobacco (Adams *et al.*, 2009; Sulkunen *et al.*, 2019). And in some places, such as Macao and the US state of Nevada, government dependence on gambling profits is far greater still. In Britain we were given clear insight into Government reliance on gambling income when the Treasury insisted that the reduction in FOBT maximum stake, that so many had been arguing for on customer protection and health grounds, would need to wait for two years until the loss of revenue it anticipated from the change could be compensated for in some other way (in the end public pressure and a Minister's resignation persuaded Government to act more quickly: see Chapter 1).

Whatever happens to the money government raises through gambling – whether a smaller or larger part goes towards 'good causes' or the prevention and treatment of gambling problems and what proportion 'disappears' into general government coffers, which also varies by jurisdiction – the proportion of gambling profits which governments take turns out to vary considerably. Drawing on a revealing study (Chambers, 2011) which compared gambling regimes based on how much revenue gambling produced for governments of different countries, Sulkunen and colleagues (2019) arrived at the estimates shown in Table 2.1.

Generally, as would be expected, countries such as the USA and Australia, with the greater availability of gambling and higher per capita spend on gambling, are those where it contributes more to the public purse. They were mostly countries which the study classified as having liberal welfare state regimes. There are some notable exceptions, however. Some such regimes are also very liberal when it comes to gambling. One example is the US state of Nevada, with its global renown as a gambling destination, where gambling companies are taxed at an unusually low rate (between 3.5 and 6.75% of profits) and are not required to contribute to public funds directly. The most notable exception is the UK, however, where Governments in the modern era of gambling policy have deliberately sought to create a regime that is attractive to gambling companies. Sulkunen *et al.* calculated an estimated contribution of gambling to UK state funds equivalent to 0.5% of the annual national state budget. In absolute terms that is, of course, a huge amount of money, but it is significantly lower than many other EU countries where public revenue from gambling they estimated to average 1.3% of state budgets. That is despite annual per capita gambling losses being similar to Britain's (as in Italy) or substantially less than Britain's (as in France and Germany).

TABLE 2.1 Size of public revenue from gambling in a number of countries (estimates in Sulkunen *et al.*, 2019, pp 150–1)

	Public revenue from gambling (as % of state budget)
Australia	7.8
USA	2.3
Canada	2.2
Finland	2.0
Italy	2.0
Sweden	1.8
France	1.7
Germany	1.6
Norway	0.6
UK	0.5

Which branches of Government?

A question which may sound bureaucratic and uninteresting, but which in reality is of the utmost importance, is that of where in government responsibility for gambling lies. The responsible ministry varies from country to country, no doubt reflecting government priorities and interests. In the UK, in line with the relatively prohibitionist policy of that era and concern about gambling and crime, gambling fell under the purview of the Home Office for most of the 20th century. It was the Home Office which had set up the Gambling Review Body (GRB) whose recommendations led to the liberalising 2005 Gambling Act. But by the time the GRB finished its work, it was required to report not to the Home Office but to the Department for Culture, Media and Sport (DCMS), now to be the lead Government department for gambling, a move which illustrated the way Government thinking on gambling had shifted. This highly significant change was scarcely noticed at the time and never received much media attention. It did not go unremarked by the GRB itself, however:

> We can readily accept that gambling is part of the leisure industry and that it would be appropriate for DCMS to sponsor it. However our concern has been with the regulation of gambling and, among other things, with the prevention of crime and harm to the vulnerable. That would appear to fall squarely with the responsibilities of the Home Office.
>
> (GRB, 2001, para 34.4)

Needless to say, a government department responsible for, among other things, leisure and sport, provides the industry with a more reliable governmental ally than a department concerned with crime and security. In the case of alcohol, responsibility for licencing shifted at the same time from the Home Office to DCMS, but other relevant departments, notably the Department of Health, are also much involved in alcohol policy, and there has been at least some attempt in that case to formulate a cross-department Government strategy. That is not the case for gambling. The Department of Health has been notably absent from British gambling policy discussions. These arrangements speak volumes about how gambling is seen by Government – more as a matter of sport and leisure than as a matter of public health. As I write, there are some welcome signs that this might be changing as part of the new backlash against uncontested gambling expansion.

Spain is another country where the controlling ministry, Finance in Spain's case, has had little coordination with other relevant ministries such as Health (Becoña & Becoña, 2018). In other countries such arrangements are often highly complicated. France is a good example: a largely state-owned monopoly controls the national and other lotteries, supervised by the Finance Ministry; casinos are in private hands, regulated by the Interior Ministry; and horse racing gambling is organised separately under the Agriculture Ministry, as it is in a number of other countries also.

Things are managed differently in different Scandinavian governments. In Sweden, the state-owned company Svenska Spel is controlled by the Ministry of Enterprise and Innovation. In Norway, the state-owned company Norsk Tipping is owned by the Ministry of Culture, and the Ministry of Agriculture and Food owns Norsk Rikstote, a foundation in charge of running tote betting. The Gaming Authority in Denmark, on the other hand, comes under the Ministry of Taxation. Lotteries in Iceland are operated under licences given by the Ministry of Justice and Ecclesiastical Affairs. The Finnish state-owned lottery and betting monopoly is regulated by the Ministry of Internal Affairs, while gambling revenues are redistributed through the Ministry of Education and Culture, Ministry of Health and Social Affairs, and Ministry of Agriculture. Unlike in the UK, the Finnish Ministry of Social Affairs and Health has a permanent consulting role on gambling harm prevention. Further complication arises in federal countries. In some, such as Mexico, Brazil and Russia, gambling is a federal matter. In others such as Australia, the USA, Canada, Switzerland and Germany, the states or provinces have the greater authority (Sulkunen *et al.*, 2019).

The wider web of dependencies

Industry and government are the two main *Gambling Establishment* partners and are often closer than they should be. *The Times* in February 2016 revealed the excessive amount of hospitality the minister responsible for gambling in Britain received from the industry between 2010 and 2012 and the apology MP Philip Davies – chair of the All Party Parliamentary Group for Betting and Gaming – had to make after not declaring hospitality from one of the biggest betting companies. Commentators on modern gambling in other parts of the world have seen something similar. In Australia, for example, there have been warnings about the rise of Big Gambling, the increasingly powerful 'industry-state gambling complex' (Markham & Young, 2014a). But the compact of organisations that become dependent on gambling profits and may become partners extends far wider. It forms:

> an extensive web of dependencies between gamblers, game providers, public authorities and the beneficiaries – associations and other institutions that deliver services and support for good causes on the basis of money coming from gamblers . . . a byzantine web of interests.
>
> (Sulkunen *et al.*, 2019, p 7)

It is not only governments and their employees and politicians who become complicit in the growth of gambling and the harm it causes. Bodies that have been relied upon to support liberalisation and to oppose further regulation of gambling in Britain include financial institutions and advertising authorities such as PricewaterhouseCoopers, mentioned earlier, and the UK's Committee of Advertising Practice and Broadcast Committee of Advertising Practice (CAP and BCAP) (see Chapter 8).

The research and academic community and service providers are also drawn into a web of dependencies on gambling (Adams, 2016; Orford, 2011). The industry link may be undisguised, as in Hong Kong where the HK University Faculty of Medicine shares a building with the HK Jockey Club Clinical Research Centre, but in most cases is more or less disguised, only advertised in discreetly placed logos or acknowledgements at the end of reports. In such cases the link may be just as threatening to the independence of a health-promoting organisation which is funded from the profits of an industry which promotes and sells the very products which have brought the organisation's patients to its door. The National Problem Gambling Clinic in London, to all appearances part of the state-provided National Health Service but in fact funded out of the levy on the gambling industry, is an example. The way that levy is administered by a third party, the charity GambleAware, is an example of something else that is very common, namely the setting up by government of various 'mediating' arrangements whereby industry profits are disbursed indirectly, giving the impression that the resources received are more independent of industry than is really the case. The conflicts of interest which inevitably arise make it less likely that those who manage and work in collaborating organisations will feel free to speak out against what the industry is doing or to champion any policy changes which might reduce industry profits.

'Partnership' is something that the industry is keen to be seen promoting. As Adams (2016) puts it, 'It repositions industry organizations away from being seen as self-seeking and profit-driven . . . to being seen more as defenders of public good alongside other equally public-spirited organizations'. Image is important for the industry, and others may be induced to see such collaboration as acceptable, even desirable. Such collaboration is not one of equally powerful partners, however. Adams' book about the risks of collaborating with industries that purvey addictive products like gambling is entitled *Moral Jeopardy* in reference to the way in which accepting some of the proceeds of selling such products, much of which should rightly be seen as 'addiction surplus', conflicts with an organisation's mission which may include treating or preventing gambling addiction. This creates a conflict of interest, and conflicts with other organisations in the same field and even within the organisation, and risks jeopardising the organisation's credibility.

The fraught issue of the dependence of gambling research on the proceeds of gambling is one that we shall look at more closely later. In Chapter 8 we will examine the lack of research funding that is truly independent of industry influence, the prominence in the field of researchers who have received substantial industry funding, and the ways in which industry funding influences the choice of research topics which receive most support and the ways in which research findings are interpreted.

Conclusion: the Gambling Establishment

By the expression the *Gambling Establishment* I mean first and foremost the industry which sells gambling, an industry which is diverse, now enormous in size and global in its scope. But it also includes a range of allies, governments and others who are colluding with this expansionist industry (see Figure 2.1). In Britain this consists of, amongst others, the Government department – now called Digital, Culture, Media and Sport – that leads on the subject, the Gambling Commission which is the body that regulates gambling, a body that advises them called the Advisory Board for Safer Gambling (ABSG, until 2019 called the Responsible Gambling Strategy Board, RGSB), and GambleAware, an industry-supported body that collects and spends the levy for treatment, prevention and research which is voluntarily donated by the industry.

The history of GambleAware is telling. It is the rebranded name of what was until 2017 the Responsible Gambling Trust (RGT), set up in 2012 as an unashamedly 'industry-led' body with the recent chair of the Association of British Bookmakers

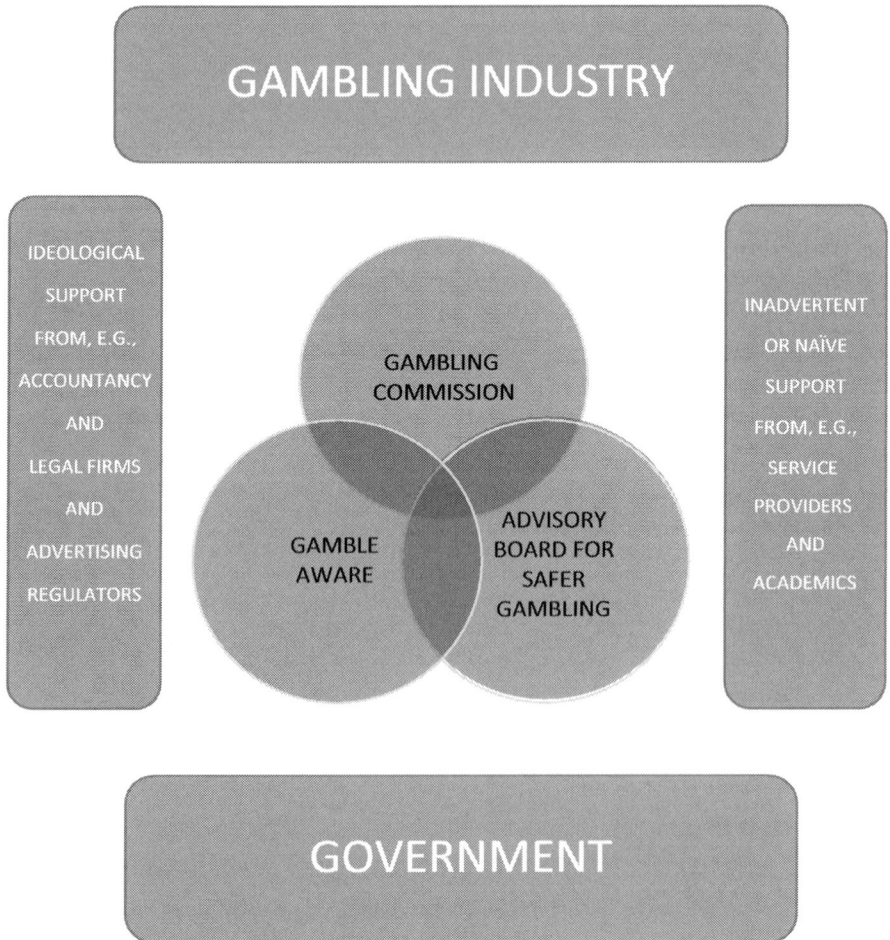

FIGURE 2.1 The British Gambling Establishment

as board chair and gambling industry representatives in half of the trustee positions. It came into being after the much more industry-independent Responsible Gambling Fund, which the Gambling Commission had recommended setting up, announced that they 'were unable to operate with the degree of independence consistent with their governance documents and their duty under charity law', and the system for trying to assure some independence in disbursing the industry levy funds broke down. The RGT was essentially an industry Social Aspects and Public Relations Organisation (a SAPRO: Babor, 2009), which like other such organisations – the alcohol industry Portman Group is another – favours the least industry-challenging harm reduction strategies such as public awareness campaigns and a focus on youth gambling and on individual gambling behaviour – 'measures that on the surface appear to address harm while at the same time posing negligible threat to the real drivers of consumption' (Adams, 2016). Despite its attempt at rebranding, GambleAware retains the industry-favourable positions consistent with its history. It failed, for example, to support the call to reduce the maximum FOBT stake size. Notably, however, neither the RGSB nor the Gambling Commission – their chief *Gambling Establishment* partners – joined the welter of expert and media opinion calling clearly for the stake size to be reduced.

Colluding, if only inadvertently, with these bodies which make up the core of the British *Gambling Establishment* are those that form the wider network of organisations, agencies and individuals who are to some degree dependent on gambling proceeds or who have been taken in by Establishment rhetoric about the place of modern commercial gambling in society. It is to that powerful Establishment ideology that we turn in the following chapter.

Notes

1 The Gambling Commission (2019a) reports a GGY (gross gambling yield: the amount retained by operators after the payment of winnings but before the deduction of the costs of the operation) for Britain for 2017–18 of £14.5 billion. That covers all gambling licenced by the Commission but underestimates the total of all legal British gambling because it excludes gambling provided in pubs, clubs, working men's clubs or family entertainment centres licenced by local authorities.
2 Quotes are taken from the meeting transcript; speakers may not have had the opportunity to check and make any necessary corrections.

3
THE ESTABLISHMENT DISCOURSE

Five ways we were told how to think about gambling

In the modern era, the massive legalised gambling industry wields power of several different kinds. For a start, it is of sufficient size and clout to be able to have its way with governments by lobbying hard, offering things that governments need and threatening to take business elsewhere if conditions are unfavourable. This is naked exercise of power, but it is perfectly legal. Indeed, it is encouraged in a free globalised market and is promoted by trade agreements that welcome competition and penalise anything that looks like restriction on free enterprise. But it operates largely out of sight of the majority of citizens whose lives may, nevertheless, be deeply affected by the increased availability of the potentially dangerous activities which new forms of gambling represent.

British Governments have been strongly criticised for allowing industry to have too much influence on public health policy. That was particularly true of the coalition Government of the early 2010s whose Public Health Responsibility Deal legitimised the role of industry in UK public health policy in an unprecedented way. Although it is the activities of the alcohol industry that have attracted more atten- tion, the same is undoubtedly true in the case of gambling. In fact, it is somewhat worse in the gambling case because, at least until recently, the connection between gambling and public health has had less media attention and the industry has been able to pursue its interests with less public scrutiny. Because of the control that the *Gambling Establishment* holds over the gambling research agenda (see Chapter 8), there has been no research on how the gambling industry uses its power to influence Government policy. That is not so true in the alcohol field where a group from the University of York and the London School of Hygiene and Tropical Medicine is just one of a number that have been busy analysing how industry wields its power with Government (McCambridge *et al.*, 2018; Savell *et al.*, 2016).

Lobbying by the industry has been found to be extensive. Industry actors engage with Members of Parliament of all parties, civil servants, Ministers,

Shadow Ministers and special advisers; they enjoy considerable access to poli-cymakers, being granted regular meetings, benefiting from extensive informal personal contact with Government, and being consulted informally both before and after official policy consultations. As David Cameron said before he became Prime Minister, 'We all know how it works. The lunches, the hospitality, the quiet word in your ear, the ex-ministers and ex-advisers for hire, helping big business find the right way to get its way' (*The Telegraph*, 2010).

But power is most effectively exercised, often without debate or even recog-nition that power is involved at all, if the status quo of increased and increasing liberalisation can be accepted by all concerned, particularly by consumers and the general public. If powerful interests can control the way people think and talk about gambling, their power is even better secured. It is a question of get-ting people to accept the 'discourses' (Lukes, 2005) which support their position. Charles Livingstone and Richard Woolley of the Department of Health Science in the Faculty of Medicine at Monash University are amongst those who have most clearly recognised this. They refer to what they call a 'comfortable orthodoxy' supporting the current unsatisfactory arrangements regarding electronic gambling machines (EGMs) in Australia. Discourses, they explained, are part of 'an active process of entrenching ways of speaking or writing about a topic such as gambling and organising knowledge and understanding about it'. As they say, so powerful is the comfortable orthodoxy and the discourses which support it, that 'It is difficult to engage with any field other than through the terms and arguments that define what can be said about it' (Livingstone & Woolley, 2007).

I know exactly what they mean by that, because I have experienced it at first hand. I have been to many meetings and conferences where gambling has been discussed, and I know how difficult it is, when all around you are using certain terms and catchphrases and making certain assumptions about the subject under discussion, to talk a different language based on a different set of assumptions. Trying to persuade us all to think about the subject in a certain way is tantamount to exerting power over us. This is a form of mental power in which ideas exert the leverage. It is all the more effective because it masquerades as something that is innocent and benign, quite different from what we think of as power (Lukes, 2005; Orford, 2013). Even though, as I shall argue, the ideas promoted are quite crude and on careful reflection easily dismissed, they are powerful if repeated often enough and supported by otherwise powerful interests and organisations. If successful, this amounts to nothing less than a form of thought control.

Nobel Prize–winning economist and once Chief Economist at the World Bank, Joseph Stiglitz (2013), is just one of a number of prominent figures who have rec-ognised the crucial importance of the intellectual framework under which policy is made and practised. He writes of the process of capturing the mindset of regu-lators, something he calls 'cognitive capture'. The same point about the power of a system of accepted ideas is made by British journalist and broadcaster Owen Jones (2015) in his book *The Establishment and How They Get Away With It*. As he rightly says, it is not 'bad' individuals with power that are the problem: 'It is the system – the Establishment – that is the problem, not the individuals who comprise it'. Writing specifically about consumption products like alcohol and gambling that are dangerous to public health, Peter Adams (2016) also, in his book *Moral Jeopardy*, talks of the 'knowledge chain' as one of the most powerful chains of industry influence on policymakers, particularly on government officials whose role is 'central in compiling, summarizing, analysing and synthesizing the current state of knowledge'.

The modern gambling market offers a splendid example of what these perceptive writers are talking about; that is, the way language is used to support certain positions and hence to serve certain interests. In the case of a legal but dangerous form of consumption such as gambling, it is now corporate interests which are served by the dominant discourse. When examined more closely, this commanding discourse turns out to be composed of a number of strands. I suggest that the discourse that has been allowed to dominate Establishment thinking about the legal, commercially supplied 'product' which is gambling comprises at least the following five elements shown in Figure 3.1 (and see Orford, 2011).

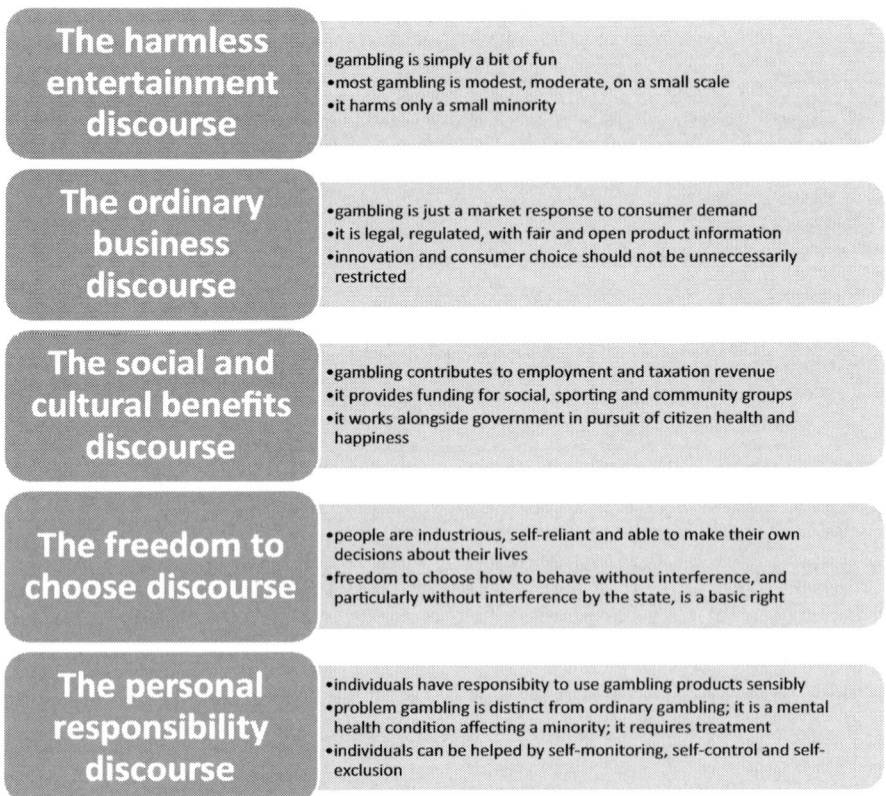

The harmless entertainment discourse	• gambling is simply a bit of fun • most gambling is modest, moderate, on a small scale • it harms only a small minority
The ordinary business discourse	• gambling is just a market response to consumer demand • it is legal, regulated, with fair and open product information • innovation and consumer choice should not be unneccessarily restricted
The social and cultural benefits discourse	• gambling contributes to employment and taxation revenue • it provides funding for social, sporting and community groups • it works alongside government in pursuit of citizen health and happiness
The freedom to choose discourse	• people are industrious, self-reliant and able to make their own decisions about their lives • freedom to choose how to behave without interference, and particularly without interference by the state, is a basic right
The personal responsibility discourse	• individuals have responsibity to use gambling products sensibly • problem gambling is distinct from ordinary gambling; it is a mental health condition affecting a minority; it requires treatment • individuals can be helped by self-monitoring, self-control and self-exclusion

FIGURE 3.1 Five elements of the Gambling Establishment discourse

Gambling is a harmless form of leisure activity and entertainment, just a bit of fun – the harmless entertainment discourse

This represents one of the main ways of thinking which gambling promoters would like us to sign up to. It has become one of the most powerful elements bolstering support for removing restrictions on the provision of gambling and resisting calls for regulations to control the more dangerous forms of modern gambling. Simple and innocuous though it sounds, this apparently unassailable message hides within it a number of points which are far from indisputable. There are several related components to this way of thinking. Let us try to unpack it. One component, which representatives of the gambling industry are particularly keen to promote, is the idea of gambling as simply a bit of fun. It is something people are prepared to pay for, much as they are prepared to pay for other forms of entertainment. If widely and uncritically accepted, this notion of gambling as, first and foremost, fun, would pave the way for virtually unlimited growth and innovation in the commercial provision of gambling. Of course there would be regulation, but not too much since it would be no job of governments to interfere with people's fun.

In chapters 4 and 5 I shall argue that the nature of gambling, particularly in its modern forms, makes it very different from ordinary kinds of fun. It is not at all like paying a fixed sum of money in return for a clearly advertised, known entertainment of fixed length or size. It is about risking money on an uncertain outcome in the hope of making a larger sum of money. In the modern era of liberalisation, commercial gambling has deviated further and further from the simple fun and entertainment model.

The harmless entertainment discourse is a key element of the influential academic *Reno Model* of gambling and problem gambling, so-called because it originated at a meeting held in Reno in the 1990s. It was then set out in four key publications between 2004 and 2015 (Blaszczynski *et al.*, 2004, 2008, 2011; Collins *et al.*, 2015) and was welcomed by the industry, governments and regulators. It 'gave the appearance of an industry and government with a social conscience' whilst 'obscuring the influence of other factors such as deceptive and misleading gambling products' (Hancock & Smith, 2017) and without challenging gambling profits. A review of the Reno Model's influence clearly identified as one of its key elements the assumption that gambling is a legal, regulated form of entertainment or recreation which harms only a small number of players. It emphasised 'fair and open' product information and education about gambling as entertainment. Alternative academic models such as 'total consumption theory', a long-established and supported public health model (Sulkunen *et al.*, 2019) which sees the amount of problem consumption of products such as gambling or alcohol as a reflection of the total amount of consumption in the whole population, have been strongly and consistently opposed by the relevant industries who favour an approach which focuses on particular high risk groups or behaviour patterns (Adams, 2016).

Because of the expertise afforded to scientists, establishment-supporting academic models, such as the Reno Model, constitute a significant part of the system and constitute one of the most important ways in which companies dealing in potentially dangerous products try to co-opt scientists (Babor, 2009). In the case of the Reno Model, this co-option appears to have gone beyond the exchange of ideas. Drawing on publicly available sources, Hancock and Smith (2017) exposed the 'significant industry funding' received by four key Reno paper authors, including Collins' £100,000 a year support from casino companies for the Centre for the Study of Gambling at the University of Salford in England. Indeed the second Reno Model paper was originally prepared for the Australian Gaming Council, the main administrative body for the gambling industry in Australia.

In the UK, the Amusement Caterers' Association, giving evidence to the Betting, Lotteries, and Gaming Royal Commission of 1949–51, was already in the business of using language effectively to control how modern gambling was to be thought of. Machine gambling was a 'wholesome entertainment that is perfectly innocuous', they claimed. To this day the gambling machine industry maintains the idea that their customers play electronic gambling machines (EGMs) for entertainment. For many years now we have referred euphemistically to premises on our highstreets that house banks of gambling machines as 'amusement arcades'. The regulatory bureaucracy now refers to them as 'adult entertainment centres'. Such attempts at thought control go on in all countries that have struggled with the issue of regulating EGMs. But in Britain it is worse. As noted in the previous chapter, British children, unlike children anywhere else, are permitted to play EGMs, requiring low stakes and offering small prizes but in all other respects just like other EGMs. Tradition has been allowed to grow up that these machines, referred to in law as B4 machines, should hardly be seen as gambling at all but rather as 'amusements' to be found in 'family entertainment centres', a traditional part of the family day out.

Most gambling, the *Gambling Establishment* says, is modest, moderate, on a small scale. This is the other, 'harmless', strand to the harmless entertainment discourse. People like me are out to spoil other people's fun, they say. We are portrayed as anti-gambling, latter-day prohibitionists. Times have changed, we are told. Gambling is no longer to be thought of as immoral or harmful. Its appropriate connotations are now those of sport, leisure, even culture. Remember that the relatively new Department for Culture, Media and Sport (DCMS), to which the British Government transferred lead responsibility for gambling in the late 1990s, was dubbed the Ministry of Fun by its first Secretary of State. As much effort is devoted by the *Gambling Establishment* towards arguing for the harmlessness of modern gambling products as towards any of the components of the pro-gambling discourse. In the process of defending the innocence of the products, they pick and interpret evidence to suit their case. The dangers inherent in modern forms of gambling are minimised. Much of the following chapters constitutes an attempt to balance the argument. Modern gambling is dangerous for individuals (Chapter 6) and for their families, communities and society generally (Chapter 7). Not everyone is harmed, it is true, but to claim that it is harmless is a distortion of the truth. The harmless entertainment discourse is particularly misleading. It needs to be challenged.

Forms of gambling are products or commodities just like any other, and their provision is just like any other form of legitimate business – the ordinary business discourse

Hand in hand with the language of harmless leisure entertainment goes the just-an-ordinary-business discourse – the idea that gambling products are ordinary commodities like any other. The Australian commentators Livingstone and Woolley (2007) referred to this as the discourse of 'Business as Usual', which represents gambling as just a market response to consumer demand. It rests on a conception of individual players as free-choosing, well-informed consumers based on the idea of consumer sovereignty and the idea that it is what the consumer wants that in the end determines what goods and services are provided. In its strong form it denies the influence of supply-side forces in constituting the market, implying that EGM gambling consumption simply reflects consumer wants. That, Livingstone and Woolley argue, is a gross oversimplification of the way in which markets are shaped, leaving out of account what they call the four Ps – product, price, promotion and place.

The ordinary business discourse was explicit in what the responsible Home Office minister said at the time when the Gambling Review Body was set up in Britain in December 1999:

> Much of our current gambling legislation is over 30 years old. Social attitudes have changed and the law is fast being overtaken by technological developments. The Government wants to get rid of unnecessary burdens on business, while maintaining protections necessary in the public interest.
>
> (Gaming Board, 2000, p 3)

In the subsequent Government proposals for legislation set out in its cleverly titled document, *A Safe Bet for Success*, the discourse of ordinary, not-to-be-restricted business predominated. For example, it was proposed to remove 'unnecessary barriers to customer access to gambling'; that 'gambling products [would be] more visible and accessible'; that gambling debts would for the first time be enforceable by law 'like other consumer contracts'; that casino operators would be freed from the existing controls which 'unnecessarily discourage innovation and restrict customer choice'; and that there was an aspiration that Britain would be a 'world leader' in online gambling. In summary, gambling was to be seen as 'an important industry in its own right, meeting the legitimate desires of many millions of people and providing many thousands of jobs', 'creat[ing] a more open and competitive gambling sector. . . [giving] better choice for consumers and enhanced opportunities for business both in the UK and abroad' (Department for Culture, Media and Sport, 2002, chapter 4). The message could not be clearer. If you ever thought that gambling held dangers for the unsuspecting and should not therefore be subject to the free market, you needed to be told in no uncertain terms that your thinking was outdated. Get modern. Join the new world of unrestricted access to consumer entertainment goods, of which gambling was one.

Around the same time, when the tax law changed, heralding the introduction of the Fixed Odds Betting Terminals – the *fob-tees* or 'roulette machines' – to British highstreet betting shops, the then Financial Secretary to the Treasury, Paul Boateng, said the changes heralded a new era for British betting. It would see Britain's betting industry become a world leader in the international betting market, and, 'Our reforms mean punters will get tax-free betting, bookmakers will see increased turnover and government revenues will share in the benefits' (The Guardian, 2001).

This ordinary commodity discourse is prominent whenever governments put their weight behind the expansion of commercial gambling. It was very evident when the Singapore Government decided that for financial reasons it would turn its back on its leaders' and citizens' previous opposition to casinos (da Cunha, 2010). It was equally clear in statements made by the commission set up by the South African Government which paved the way for large numbers of casinos in that country. The commission's philosophy was that 'market forces will be the major determining factor with regard to the allocation and distribution of casino . . . licences' (Sallaz, 2009). The same arguments have been much heard in Australia, where the machine design industry has been particularly vigorous. The Australasian Gaming Machine Manufacturers Association (2007), when making submissions to the New South Wales and Australian Governments, argued against restrictions which would be inconsistent with 'an open technology environment' or interfere with them having 'the freedom and flexibility to expend major research and development resources, to innovate, to develop new products.'

I hope to be able to show in the rest of this book that, contrary to the business-as-usual discourse, gambling is no ordinary commodity. It never has been. Everyone knows, and has always known, that gambling is dangerous. What is not always appreciated is just how much more dangerous gambling has become. New laws and regulations based on the discourse of gambling as a commodity like any other have given the industry the green light to innovate and to sell us ever more dangerous products. Indeed, why would it not do so? If governments tell it that it is in the business mainstream, why would it not do what good businesses do – innovate and expand? The result is that we are exposed to greater danger.

Gambling enhances the life of communities economically and in terms of leisure opportunities and cultural life in general – the social and cultural benefits discourse

Reinforcing the ordinary business discourse is another which says that gambling enhances the life of communities or a whole nation not just economically but also

The complexity of the motivation to gamble is illustrated by one of the fullest studies of the subject, carried out in New Zealand. Following a comprehensive review of earlier work and the conducting of a large number of open-ended interviews and focus groups with gamblers, professionals and family members, a questionnaire was devised and administered to over 300 adult gamblers. They were asked to say which of a number of statements reflected the reasons why they started to gamble and the reasons why they had continued to gamble regularly (Clarke *et al.*, 2006). That careful study, which used a good balance of different methods, shows that gambling behaviour is determined by an interaction of different influences. Some of these are things that people bring with them to the activity. Others are characteristics of the activity being offered, the setting in which it is offered and how it is offered.

Consistent with other studies of gamblers' motivations to gamble (e.g. Binde, 2013; Wardle *et al.*, 2011), it comes across clearly that the hope of winning money was the reason most frequently given both for starting to gamble and for continuing to gamble regularly – reaching almost 100% of agreement on the part of the gamblers who took part. Almost equally endorsed were reasons to do with seeking excitement, entertainment and socialising, with escaping from stress and boredom becoming more important as reasons for continuing regular gambling.

But alongside these economic, personal and social reasons, the friendliness of the gambling products themselves, the attractiveness of the gambling environment and the way gambling was promoted were seen as equally important. One of the main themes identified amongst reasons for starting to gamble was what the authors of this report referred to as 'the 4 As' – the advertising, availability, accessibility and abundance of various forms of gambling activity. For example, the large majority agreed about the importance of the places where the respondent socialised having gambling facilities; advertisements encouraging the respondent to think he or she could win; having easy access to gambling activities and to money machines; and liking the sound and excitement of gaming venues.

This chapter will focus on how gambling is advertised and promoted in the modern era of gambling liberalisation, leaving to the following chapter consideration of the nature of modern gambling itself and of gambling venues.

Bombarded by gambling advertising

One of the most obvious things the 2005 Gambling Act did for Britain was to ease many of the gambling advertising restrictions, particularly on advertising gambling products on television. There followed an explosion in gambling marketing; resources devoted to advertising gambling since then have been huge. Ofcom (2013) reported an increase of 1,444% in gambling advertisements between 2005 and 2012. Gambling's share of the advertising market grew from 0.5% to 4.1% over the period. According to the Advertising Association, which represents the advertising industry, about £150 million was spent on gambling advertising in Britain in 2010, most on sports gambling, lotteries and bingo. William Hill alone had a in terms of leisure opportunities and cultural life in general. National lotteries have perhaps the best claim on that account. As in other countries, the National Lottery in Britain, run by a monopoly provider under Government licence, has been heavily promoted by emphasising the contributions it makes to national 'good causes'. But such claims have not been confined to national lotteries. They have been made in countries around the world whenever new casino complexes have been proposed. Much was made of the way in which Britain's first regional casino, if it came to Blackpool, would rejuvenate this once iconic English sea-side resort. The new casino developments in Singapore were billed as part of the country's attempt to style itself as a 'Renaissance city of Asia', the 'Monaco of the East' (da Cunha, 2010). The South African commission report opened by stating that gambling policy must advance 'social upliftment and economic development' (Sallaz, 2009). Similar claims have been made elsewhere, for example at Niagara Falls in Canada, in Atlantic City in the USA and in Hamilton in New Zealand. After the Hamilton casino opened, according to the Waikato Times (1997), 'Hamilton is no longer a boring provincial city. It's a go-ahead place, a metropolitan city which offers its populace a choice in what they can do'.

This extends the business-as-usual discourse by making it look as if providing gambling commercially is not just good for profits and taxes because it is selling a desired product but also a general societal good. In modern parlance, the suggestion is that it contributes positively to a nation's cultural and economic capital. Chapter 7 will question this claim that gambling in its modern commercial forms is good for society. As we saw in Chapter 1, most citizens actually believe the opposite.

The way gambling was portrayed as having positive social and economic effects for the community was also one of the main themes identified in a 2016 analysis of the prevailing official thinking about gambling in Australia. The benefits, often mentioned in relevant documents, included entertainment, employment, taxation revenue, and funding for social, sporting and community groups. Gambling was also portrayed as beneficial to the local community, for example by creating social capital through volunteering and by gambling venues working with charity groups and others from the local community. A related basic theme positioned gambling as a key part of Australian cultural heritage. Clubs Australia, for example, claimed in 2012 that gambling was 'an integral part of the Australian culture', justifying this by stating that '70 percent of Australians participate in some form of gambling each year' (Miller *et al.*, 2016).

Peter Adams from New Zealand calls this the 'public-good' chain of industry influence on policy – the others are the political chain and the knowledge chain. He refers, for example, to gambling company donations to charities such as Children with Leukaemia and Breakthrough Breast Cancer. In the New Zealand context such 'gifts' announced as philanthropy, he suggests, are a 'masquerade' since the main purposes are 'positive image building . . . cementing relations of obligation with opinion leaders, promoting organizational dependency, silencing critics . . . and establishing legitimacy in health policy debates' (Adams, 2016). He cites the Lion Foundation, a New Zealand–wide gambling machine trust, which proclaims its contribution to community causes as if this is freely given when in fact the country's regulatory framework was set up to provide benefits to communities as a central purpose and the legislation requires them to do this, even specifying the amounts to be donated and which groups are eligible for funding. Hence, what are made out to be donations should really be seen as resembling a form of taxation rather than philanthropy.

There is an important sub-plot to the social and cultural benefits discourse which is about partnership. The latter is something that the gambling industry emphasises repeatedly. This was recognised in the analysis of Reno Model documents (Hancock & Smith, 2017): that key responsible gambling stakeholders have similar goals and need to work collaboratively. Far from being seen as a danger to the public good, commercial gambling should be seen as contributing positively to it. It works alongside government in its pursuit of citizen health and happiness, not in opposition to it. This is an all-important element of the Establishment discourse because it positions the industry as a partner in the pursuit of the common good rather than as a body with a conflict of interests. It follows that the industry should have a prominent place in forums where public health is discussed and debated, rather than be excluded from them. From this perspective, government, the public health community and industry should be seen as partners, not adversaries.

Citizens should be free to choose how to use their leisure time, including being free to gamble as they wish – the freedom to choose discourse

The freedom to choose how to behave without interference, and particularly without interference by the state, is another key element in this powerful amalgam of discourses. It is difficult to gainsay. Prohibition has a bad reputation and is generally unpopular. A belief in freedom as a cornerstone of the concept of the rights of citizens in free countries is deeply held. The charge that one is a supporter of the 'nanny state' is one of the most difficult to refute. The appeal of this discourse is nothing new. When temperance sentiments were strong in Britain at the end of the Victorian era and the Anti-Gambling League almost succeeded in getting horse race betting banned altogether, the secretary of the Anti-Puritan League complained to the Home Secretary about the 'grandmotherly interference of self-righteous faddists' and 'meddlesome attempts . . . to interfere with the national sports and pastimes of the people' (Miers, 2004).

Almost a hundred years later in his book *Gambling and the Public Interest*, a basic Reno Model text, British gambling professor Peter Collins (2003), who worked closely with the gambling industry in South Africa, opined that 'interfering with people's freedom of choice to protect them from harming themselves goes against and goes beyond the legitimate role of government in a free society', and that 'government has no business interfering with the exchanges of goods and services between willing buyers and willing sellers'. The South African gambling commission report said the state should 'allow as little interference as possible with the gambler's freedom to gamble' (Sallaz, 2009). This plea is widely heard, nowhere more so than in Australia and New Zealand. The chair of the Gaming Association in New Zealand declared, 'Gambling is part and parcel of life in New Zealand and Australia. Our people are industrious, self-reliant and able to make their own decisions about their lives' (Adams, 2008).

The anti-government interference strand to the freedom to choose discourse is, in practice, of greatest importance. Reviewers of the Reno Model, Hancock and Smith (2017), believe that the model stems from a libertarian ideology which 'disdains government regulations that diminish individual liberty and autonomy . . . freedom of choice, gambling as entertainment' and views the gambling industry as similar to other legal industries but unfairly heavily taxed and over-regulated. It is not just the freedom of the individual that is being protected here but also, and perhaps more significantly for policy, the freedom of the industry from government interference. It is notable that the British Government, as it announced its long-delayed decision to interfere by reducing the maximum stake on the FOBTs, felt it necessary to make it clear that their intention was to continue to take a back seat when it came to gambling, giving the industry a central position. It said, 'we want to see industry, regulator and charities continue to drive the social responsibility agenda, to ensure that all is being done to protect players without the need for further Government intervention' (Department for Digital, Culture, Media and Sport, 2018).

Much of the rest of the present book constitutes an argument against this apparently inviolate dictum about freedom. In fact, it is not so difficult to challenge it. No one has ever suggested – not even the much invoked John Stuart Mill – that we should be free to do anything, however harmful it is to other people. As Hancock and Smith said about the Reno Model, it may be strong on civil liberties, but it is short on human rights and consumer protection. The questions that need to be asked are, Whose freedom is being protected by the expansion and development of commercial gambling? And, who is being harmed in the process? The latter question is taken up in Chapter 7.

Consumers have a responsibility to protect their own health and well-being, and that of others close to them, by gambling responsibly – the personal responsibility discourse

The most modern, and possibly most powerful, addition to the cluster of Establishment gambling discourses speaks of 'responsible gambling'. It sits well with notions of gambling supply and consumption as ordinary business, harmless amusement and free choice. The idea that consumers have an obligation to consume these products 'responsibly' is a concept that was widely signed up to by not only much of the gambling industry but also governments, gambling regulators and even organisations whose aims are the treatment and prevention of gambling addiction. In Britain we had a Responsible Gambling Trust (now GambleAware) and a Responsible Gambling Strategy Board (now the Advisory Board for Safer

Gambling). Official pronouncements about gambling and reports and documents on the subject have been peppered with the expression 'responsible gambling'. At first blush, this looks completely reasonable. What could there possibly be to object to in the idea that, if there is to be gambling, it should be done responsibly? However, only a little reflection on the idea, plus observation of the way it is used in practice, are needed in order to see clearly how this idea of responsible gambling serves Establishment aims of promoting an expansionist gambling industry.

The concept of responsible gambling was a public relations coup for the gambling industry and its supporters. It sounded sufficiently unproblematic to be able to fool most people most of the time. But only just below the surface its message was clear and powerful. There are those who will argue that responsible gambling refers as much to operators being responsible in the way they provide gambling. In practice, however, it emphasises the responsibility of players for their own gambling decisions and any harm that may ensue and is comparatively quiet about the responsibilities of the suppliers. The suppliers' responsibility is limited to making sure that consumers are 'informed' about the product. Hancock and Smith argue that the Reno Model, instead of proposing a reasonable balance between industry, government and individual responsibility, supports a biased focus on individual responsibility. To quote from one of the key Reno Model documents: 'Once informed about the attributes of an activity, gamblers assume the burden of gambling responsibly; they must consider the individual and social consequences of their gambling choices' (Blaszczynski *et al.*, 2011, cited by Hancock & Smith, 2017).

In the case of gambling, the idea of 'informed consumers' is problematic since much of the information – some of it highly technical – about how games operate and the odds of winning and losing are not transparent, and very few jurisdictions require that gambling operators publish odds pertaining to different games or different machines. Since the odds are necessarily stacked against the player, it could be argued that full transparency about the odds of winning and losing, combined with education about statistical probability, would be bound to undermine efforts to market gambling. We shall have much more to hear about this in chapters 4 and 5.

One of the implications of the responsible gambling discourse, interpreted to mean that the lion's share of the obligation to behave responsibly falls on the consumers, is that the large majority consume the product responsibly, leaving only a small, even 'tiny', minority who do not or cannot use the product responsibly. Statements about responsible gambling often, therefore, involve a minimising and marginalising of those thought to be at risk. Anthropologist Natasha Schüll (2012), in her book about EGMs in Las Vegas, has much to say about the gambling discourse that we were taught. She gives us numerous examples of the way in which the industry representatives she spoke to talked about the subject. She refers to this as the use of 'defence mechanisms' on the industry's part. One common defence was the familiar 'only a small minority fits the criteria for problem gambling' defence. This, 'narrow[s] the responsibility down to a small group of people that cause the problems and argu[es] that their indiscretions cannot justify restricting the freedom to gamble for the public as a whole' (Adams, 2008).

It gets much worse. There is a not so subtle implication behind the idea of responsible gambling that problem gamblers are not just a very small minority but also that this is a deviant minority who bring their deviance to their gambling. This was horribly illustrated in the submission made by the American Gaming Association (AGA) to the Australian Senate when it was considering the possibility of restrictions on the operation of gambling machines in 2008. Such restrictions, AGA argued, would 'reduce the enjoyment of the other ninety-nine per cent of people who play the gambling machines for recreation'. This small minority who threatened the enjoyment of the majority were, 'troubled people. . . [with] alarming levels. . . [of] comorbidity. . . [suggesting] a disturbing picture of the individuals who are unable to control their gambling' (AGA, 2008). This can be clearly recognised as a particularly cruel example of the unfortunately common defence of 'blaming the victim', a tactic to which the powerful all too frequently resort in defence of their exploitative activities. The South African commission report, referred to earlier, also argued that while 'normal' gamblers play for fun and risk only what they can afford to lose, a small proportion of any population suffers from 'a psychological abnormality in which they are driven by inner urges to gamble uncontrollably' (Sallaz, 2009).

The idea that only a tiny proportion of gamblers run into trouble with their gambling and that problem gambling is a comparatively negligible public health issue rests on a complete misrepresentation of the facts. Even worse is the idea – nothing less than cruel and unjust – that those who do get into trouble are most appropriately thought of as behaving irresponsibly.

Two studies that expose how the responsible gambling discourse serves establishment interests

Two studies have analysed various sources in detail in an effort to unpack the concept of responsible gambling. One, already referred to, which looked at government and gambling industry websites, television campaigns and other responsible gambling materials, was carried out in Australia. Two overriding themes were detected. One corresponded to the familiar entertainment and social and cultural benefits of gambling discourses – gambling as entertainment or recreation, gambling's positive social and economic effects, and gambling as an integral part of Australian culture. But it is the other element which is highly relevant in the context of responsible gambling. The essence of this important theme was the contrast between most ordinary gambling and problem gambling. There were a number of strands: problem gambling is rare; it is uniquely harmful, with negative consequences for the gambler and the community; it is a mental health condition; it requires counselling. It is worth quoting the summary abstract from the published paper:

Results: Documents distinguished between gambling, which was positive for the community, and problem gambling, which was portrayed as harmful and requiring medical intervention. The need for responsible gambling was emphasised in many of the documents, and reinforced by mechanisms including self-monitoring, self-control and surveillance of gamblers. *Conclusions*: Government and industry expect gamblers to behave 'responsibly', and are heavily influenced by neoliberal ideas of rational, controlled subjects in their conceptualisation of what constitutes 'responsible behaviour'. As a consequence, problem gamblers become constructed as a deviant group. This may have significant consequences for problem gamblers, such as the creation of stigma.

(Miller *et al.*, 2016, p 163)

The other study I want to mention scrutinised more closely these ideas of responsibility and control. It was a particularly thorough Swedish study based on 40 interviews conducted with key informants including representatives of gambling operators, NGOs, public authorities, care providers, gamblers themselves and journalists, as well as analysis of thousands of pages of policy documents, newspaper articles, and gambling operator and other reports (Alexius, 2017).

The language used by the author of this interesting report is social science speak, but it hits the nail on the head. It notes how 'the previous responsibility order' dominated by government taking responsibility for protecting citizens by closely controlling gambling, often prohibiting much of it, had been complemented by an increasingly 'market-embedded order'. This is a shift in where responsibility is assumed to lie, from the protective state to the market consumer, towards gamblers being viewed first as consumers and only secondly as citizens. One notable consequence has been the emergence of what the author calls 'responsibility services' now being offered to gambling consumers. A 'side-market' of online 'seatbelts and helmets' for responsible gambling tools and services has emerged – such as information, training, interactive tools and standards – with the goal of shaping and equipping consumers to better 'navigate the temptations of consumer society and make informed choices'.

An example given was the responsible gaming site offered by Svenska Spel. A content analysis suggested that, despite its representatives' claim that their site was not pointing fingers at anyone, the message being conveyed was a clear one: gambling is enjoyable only if it occurs 'in moderation'; gamblers should think and reflect and be aware. With its warm, welcoming voice supported by cartoon talk bubbles, colourful symbols and friendly figures, the site encouraged the gambler to get to know its portfolio of responsible gaming services. These included Svenska Spel's loyalty card that gave gamblers access to all its tools and the ability to view their own gambling trends over time, a gaming budget tool that helped gamblers establish a personal gambling budget in advance, and a self-test that surveyed the player's gambling habits via 20 multiple-choice questions and statements and provided a personal gambling profile accompanied by a Warning!/Caution!/OK traffic signal icon. The site also offered an advanced interactive monitoring service, Playscan, developed by Svenska Spel in 2006 in collaboration with mathematicians and psychologists with the aim of convincing customers to remain in what the project manager called the 'healthy, green gambling zone' by predicting future gambling behaviour and issuing a warning, if needed, 'while the customer is still rational and receptive'.

The division of responsibility was clear. Gamblers were informed of the risks they might be running, but the decision to reduce or stop gambling was wholly the gambler's own. Almost all the responsible gambling tools focussed on continued consumption according to the 'play in moderation!' message. This, explained the Svenska Spel CEO at the time, was a deliberate message, necessary for the state-owned company to fulfil its mission of making profits whilst being socially responsible at the same time. With the EU demanding that nationalised gambling operators demonstrate social responsibility, it became vital to 'craft a responsibility position that would grant legitimacy without having to compromise th[at] dual mission'.

What surprised the author of this report, but which I don't find so surprising, was that adherence to this responsibility order characterised by 'consumer responsibilisation', not unexpected for those involved in providing gambling, was shared by nearly all other organisations in the field. This included charity caregivers and support associations such as the Stockholm Addiction Treatment Centre, an outpatient care unit connected to Karolinska University Hospital, and the support organisation The National Association for Gambling Addicts (SBRF). As one of the social workers at the former explained, it was policy to emphasise personal responsibility, and, furthermore, the centre staff saw it as unhelpful to talk about the government's or the gambling companies' responsibility for gambling problems (Alexius, 2017, p 469):

> I think that much of the purpose of the treatment is to teach people that they can take control of their lives – that it is *their* responsibility. Many of the effective components of . . . treatment emphasize the person's own autonomy – it's *you* who decide what you want to do with your life. And no one can make that decision for you. It's *you* who shape your everyday life. So dwelling too much on things like banning games, the responsibility of the government and the gambling companies is counterproductive.

The chair of the Stockholm branch of SBRF put it this way (Alexius, 2017, p 470):

> Individual responsibility is what we stress *all the time*, I mean it's almost our first commandment, because that is what it's all about, our work. It's about getting people to take responsibility themselves. [. . .] When people show up who don't think that it's their fault that they gamble but that it's Svenska Spel's and ATG's [another Swedish gambling company's] fault, we don't have that discussion. We say: 'Get your life in order. We can't solve the other stuff here

[regulation and policy matters], but you, *yourself*, can stop playing if you're motivated enough'.

This important report demonstrates very clearly what I mean by the *Gambling Establishment* and its shared dominant discourse. Perhaps inadvertently, those who manage treatment and support services also take on board ways of thinking and talking about gambling harm which support the industry position. Where much of gambling provision is nationalised, as it has been in Sweden, or when treatment services are funded directly or indirectly by the industry, as is still the mostly the case in Britain, the collusion with industry and government discourse is most obvious, but it is ubiquitous.

As Peter Adams argues, 'both industry and governments have an interest in keeping initiatives focused primarily on the individual', with problems, when they do arise, being seen exclusively as a result of deficiencies in the behaviour of individual consumers and with the focus taken off product design, consuming environments or policy frameworks and governments' duty of care. This shift of responsibility from structural change to behaviour change is so important because it 'weakens the case for policy change; it is the consumers that need to change, not the way products are made available' (Adams, 2016).

The Gambling Establishment discourse needs to be challenged

In summary, the Establishment thinking about gambling – the official gambling discourse – was utterly transformed in the modern era of liberalised gambling. The powerful alliance of the industry and governments did its level best to get us all to think about gambling in the same way. No longer was gambling to be seen as immoral, irrational, tawdry, exploitative, a vice that a nation should be ashamed of – all, we were told, examples of worn-out narratives unsuited to modern times. Alongside the selling of their products, the gambling industry sold the ideas that their businesses were no different from any others, that the commodities they dealt in were not only harmless if used properly but were positively beneficial for individuals and communities, that the freedom of citizens to use their products as they choose is a fundamental right not to be interfered with and, perhaps most important of all, that those who do experience difficulty using these commodities are failing to show due responsibility. It is this collection of ideas, cloaking these industries in an apparel of respectability, which constitutes the Establishment Discourse. Challenging it is not easy because:

> the official discourse is ubiquitous and it is empowered; it is the voice of convention, the voice of authority, the voice of the law. . . . It shapes the language we speak and the categories we learn and use to think about the world. It is, quite simply, embedded in our culture.

That was Merrill Singer (2008, p 28) writing about the power of the commercial alcohol industry. But her words apply equally to the gambling-promoting industry. When we are constantly being fed the same collection of ideas, it is difficult to resist. But there are very good grounds for seeing things differently. The *Gambling Establishment* should not be allowed to get away with winning the intellectual argument. It needs to be challenged. And it can be.

In fact there are encouraging signs that the 'responsible gambling' argument, at least, is starting to wear thin. I am now finding myself having conversations with people who formerly would have accepted it without question but who are now less sure about it. In Melbourne, I heard from the Chief Executive of the Victorian Responsible Gambling Foundation (VRGF, funded by but operating independently of the Victorian Government). Introducing their first conference, he said that he saw Bet Regret – which aims to draw attention to the significance of the common experience of regretting having bet and lost more than one meant to or could afford – as a message that could take the place of the Responsible Gambling message about which he felt ambivalent – despite it being in the Foundation's title. Back home in the UK, the Responsible Gambling Trust has tried to rebrand itself as GambleAware and conversations with the Gambling Commission suggest that they too are becoming conscious of the downsides of the responsible gambling message. I take these as further indications of the backlash against the expansion and development of commercial gambling that is now occurring. Nevertheless, the intellectual edifice, the cognitive structure of commanding discourses, which has underpinned the modern explosion of gambling, is still very much in place. It will not be dislodged easily. As I outline in the final chapter, meaningful change in gambling policy will require replacing it with a distinctly different discourse.

It is time now to look more closely at some of the modern gambling products themselves, whose promotion and provision is underpinned by the Establishment discourses we have been looking at in this chapter. We shall start in the next chapter by looking at one of the aspects of early-21st-century gambling which people find most distasteful – gambling advertising.

4

HOW GAMBLING IS FORCIBLY ADVERTISED AND SOLD IN THE MODERN ERA

The gambling industry view is that the commercial provision of gambling is simply meeting a pre-existing need. Otherwise why would it flourish? It is to be understood as just another example of companies providing a service for which there is a market. People seem to want it. That makes it all seem plain and innocent. After all no one is forced to do anything they don't want to do. But those who have looked more closely at modern forms of gambling provision have seen it as more complicated than that. Gambling is sold rather forcibly, they point out. It has even been suggested that the 'need' for gambling, rather than pre-existing, is actually created by the way in which it is advertised and offered. Perhaps it was always so. But in the case of modern forms of gambling, the case for the need being a 'created' one is particularly strong.

How the product is supplied has an important effect on gambling motivation

To look solely at the motivation of the gambler is to take a one-sided view of what motivates gambling. It starts out with the assumption that the answer to the question of why people gamble lies with the individual. A more complete answer to the question should consider both person and product, both the buyer's individual motivation and the seller's motivation, including the way in which the product is advertised and sold to us. When it comes to dangerous forms of consumption with potential for addiction, it has been long understood that such behaviours can be attributed both to the person (P), the environment (E) and the interaction between the two (P X E). In the field of public health it has been axiomatic for years that understanding the spread of disease must take account of the infectious agent, the host and the environment. And in the field of drug addiction specifically it has long been accepted that drug use is to do with some combination of person, drug and setting (Zinberg, 1978).

total advertising spend in 2008 of €12.6 million, half of it spent on online advertising (Jones, 2017). The wide range of strategies used to market gambling includes television, radio, newspapers and magazines, large billboards and smaller adverts on buses and elsewhere, plus direct mail, official and affiliated websites, email newsletters, and third-party emails (Banks, 2014). In Australia, where commercial gambling and the amount of advertising have provoked particular concern, participants in one study spoke of being 'bombarded' by gambling advertising (Thomas *et al.*, 2012).

Content: the appeal and exaggeration of winning

When it comes to the content of gambling advertisements, one recognised international authority is the Swedish social scientist Per Binde. His observations about 'truth, deception, and imagination in gambling advertising' (2009) are among the best on the subject. They are worth spelling out in some detail. Just like in Britain, up until the 1980s the official position regarding gambling in his country was that operators were allowed only minimal promotion to passively meet demand for gambling but should do nothing to increase demand. This changed in the 1980s, as it did in Britain and elsewhere, and by 2006 the largely state-owned company Svenska Spel was spending the equivalent of around €25 million on advertising annually. As Binde said, the rise in gambling advertising is clear to everyone; it 'seems to be everywhere, flooding us from all directions'. Gambling policy was constantly debated in the Swedish media, and gambling advertising had become a politically hot issue. Several political parties, Christian organisations and other NGOs were demanding restrictions on advertising. The grounds for their demands were several – that it increases the amount of money spent on gambling as well as problem gambling, that it is morally unacceptable to promote gambling when it is known to cause harm and particularly for a state-owned gambling company to do so, and that it undermines the work ethic and encourages such ills as materialism, irrationality and social and political passivity. Binde's concern was not so much with those arguments, which he thought could be seen as a reflection of the somewhat paternalistic aspect of Swedish welfare ideology, but rather with the misleading nature of much gambling advertising.

He analysed about 250 Swedish newspaper, magazine, poster, direct mail, television and film advertisements for gambling, collected mainly in 2004. His conclusions are interesting and continue to apply to gambling advertising well beyond Sweden. For a start, advertising must capture attention and, like other advertising, he found gambling advertising used humour, huge text on billboards, celebrity endorsement and the repetition of a message over and over again in order to do this. Swedish gambling promotion included informative advertising – for example, about current jackpots, new games, financing good causes, special events and offerings. But, again in common with other forms of advertising, gambling advertising strayed well beyond the strictly informative. There were adverts which suggested that one might become rich through gambling and others suggesting that knowledge was essential for success in sports betting. Others emphasised the fun of gambling or the excitement of playing, the entertainment offered and other things pertaining to the experience and the environment.

But his main focus was on devices used to enhance the perception of the chances of winning, that being central to individuals' motives to gamble, according to his reading of the evidence, with all other personal motives being secondary to it. Virtually all gambling advertising, he found, was based on an explicit or implicit message that there is a chance of winning money. This is essentially misleading. For example, lottery advertising statements such as 'You can win a million' or 'The ticket that can transform your life', although undeniably true, overshadow the important question of how likely – or rather unlikely – a big win really is. In fact, using a variety of psychological and rhetorical devices, gambling advertising promotes the perception that there are many winners and encourages people to imagine themselves as winners while saying little about the chances of winning.

As Binde nicely put it, 'The real world with the actual minimal chances of winning a jackpot is replaced by a dreamworld dense with symbols of affluence, leisure, and pleasures'. This was done in a variety of clever ways in the Swedish adverts and is essentially the same in Britain and elsewhere. Lottery draws were broadcast to large television audiences. Happy previous winners were shown. Suggestive questions were asked such as 'What would *you* do if you won a million?', or, 'You could win one of 100 new cars – which one will be *your* choice?' The total amount of winnings was highlighted – 'A thousand million in winnings last year'. The consequences of winning rather than the probability of doing so were depicted; for example, holidaying in a tropical paradise, bundles of banknotes or participating in exclusive sports. Exaggerating the skill element in horse and other sports betting was another device commonly employed – 'The one who knows the most, wins the most', 'Become a football pool millionaire', 'Luck has nothing to do with it'.

This kind of misleading advertising is, of course, mostly perfectly legal. Any advertising which is objectively deceptive is against the law. A statement such as 'Luck has nothing to do with it', Binde points out, might be an interesting borderline case. There are conflicting views about advertising generally. A critical view sees it as deceptive and dangerous, whereas the view of the market is that it is good for companies as for consumers and for society because it is necessary for competition. Some minor deception, it is argued, is not worrying since consumers are knowledgeable, and any company that seriously deceives will hurt its own reputation. Anyway, more than 75% of Swedish people agreed that 'Nearly all advertising aims to mislead the public'.

But Binde was not so complacent. Examples of themes that he suggested were questionable because they might be seriously misleading included the following: emphasis on the sum of total winnings, statements that a player 'can' win millions or 'has a chance' to win the jackpot, emphasis on huge jackpots, suggestions that 'winning is easy', imagery of an abundance of money and attractive groups of other lottery prizes, the unrealistic depiction of how winning changes a person's life, stress on the total number of top prize-winners, and suggestions that skilled players win more money than less skilled ones in pari-mutuel games – the skill element is overestimated by players and in advertising.

Large wins are extremely rare, and focussing on this, he thought, was misleading, stimulating wishful thinking and causing overestimation of the chances of winning. It might be argued that sustaining the hope of winning is positive whether it is true or false, enriching the quality of life, but for others, he says, 'the hope of the jackpot win is desperate, born out of poverty, debt, and perhaps huge gambling losses. Such desperate hope can hardly be regarded as "enriching"'. Binde was particularly critical of vague and symbolic messages which tried to portray an association between products and brands and positive cultural and social values rather than providing information about the products.

The seductive nature of online gambling promotion

It comes as little surprise to learn about the many ways in which online providers woo their customers. Some of their methods are transparent and above board. Others are questionable, if not legally then certainly ethically. There have been a number of studies that have exposed these methods. I shall refer to three of them, two English, the third Canadian.

The first English study, which came from the International Gaming Research Unit at Nottingham Trent University, looked at online gambling from the players' perspective (McCormack & Griffiths, 2012). Interviews with online gamblers about the attractions of that way of gambling showed how effective gambling sites were in achieving their aim of giving their customers something that was difficult to resist. The overriding factor for that study's informants was, as one might expect, its convenience, the way in which the internet provided greater opportunity to gamble. It made available '24-hour gambling'. The value for money that internet gambling offered was also an important motivating factor for many. The online gambling industry has significantly lower costs and is able to offer players more competitive prices and tempting promotional offers.

Half of those interviewed said they were attracted by the offer of free bets on gambling websites. They referred to the bonuses which matched customer deposit amounts, offered a free stake to gamble with, or awarded loyalty points that could be exchanged for prizes. Some checked out many websites to find out about the free bets on offer. Inexperienced players, at poker for example, had the opportunity online to practice for free or with very small stakes in order to gain experience, neither of which would be possible at a casino. Players found it attractive that sites offered the possibility of playing for points rather than money until a player felt confident enough to play with his or her own money or to enter live tournaments. This reduced any embarrassment caused by being a novice. It has been shown, the authors of the report say, that these 'free plays' often give a false impression of the likelihood of winning because the odds are arranged to be more in the player's favour than is the case when playing for money.

The other British study I want to mention used a different methodology. It was a study conducted at Sheffield Hallam University of over 3,000 direct email online gambling promotions sent out by 67 gambling promoters (Banks, 2014). Its results support many of Binde's Swedish findings, including the portrayal of gambling as glitzy and glamorous, the frequent use of sexualised images and the emphasis on friendship and socialising with appeal to young people. Over a third tried to normalise gambling by constructing it as an everyday activity and rational consumer purchase. But the main themes were an emphasis on skill and knowledge, which were mentioned three times as often as chance or luck, and 'Winning, winning big, and winning as the only outcome of online gambling', with the actual probability of winning and 'winning big' rarely alluded to. Words such as 'gamble' or 'gambling' were avoided in favour of terms such as 'flutter', 'punt' or simply 'bet'. This 'softening of language', which has often been noted, 'disguises the use of money in gambling and distances the player from financial loss'. Meanwhile much is made of the rare big win, as in: 'A lucky lady from Yorkshire is £150,000 richer after hitting the jackpot on our Rainbow Riches slot! Could you be next to collect the pot of gold at the end of the rainbow?' 'Largely ignored', the report points out, 'are the dangerous risks that may be attached to online gambling, including the insecurity of websites, the fairness and integrity of games, underage and problem gambling, crime and victimisation, and the potential for significant financial loss'.

The Canadian study was carried out by a group of researchers from Nova Scotia (McMullan & Kervin, 2012). They analysed 71 online poker sites in great detail. The sites they looked at were representative of the different jurisdictions from which companies operated and covered relatively popular and less popular sites. Each site was examined at least twice by more than one researcher. It is worth describing the results of that carefully executed study in some detail. It provides a fascinating but alarming picture of the methods being used to draw people in.

From a technical point of view, the Canadian researchers found the majority of the sites they visited to be highly sophisticated, fast and easy to navigate. They informed customers how to get around the site, enter a competition, find a table, take a seat, open an account and interact with others, and they offered support services to manage consumer questions and problems. Nearly all provided privacy policies that customers had to accept, providing basic information about game integrity, ensuring customers that true random-number generators and sophisticated algorithms were used and audited, and issuing statements about how they combated fraud, cheating and collusion. Most sites, it was noted, went out of their way to encourage feelings that players were gambling globally. Poker Stars, for example, supported 23 languages with statements such as 'Join the world's largest poker VIP club'. A master message, as the report's authors call it, promoted on the large majority of sites, was that poker was a legitimate consumption practice that is taking place constantly, every minute of every day: 'round the clock tournament action', as Cake Poker put it. Party Poker offered 14 different tournaments, including 'Play for an Asian adventure in Macau'.

Sites used attractive colour schemes, almost two-thirds using bright, intense, bold colours to convey conviviality and to suggest that play was pleasurable, arousing and challenging. There was much use of icons, signs, human images, banners and pop-ups, with images flashing continuously routing online traffic to gambling events and encouraging players to download free software, to set up accounts quickly and to start gambling straightaway. One in 10 promoted overtly sexualised imagery. Bikini Poker, for example, featured a picture of nine women wearing bikinis that scrawled across every page of the website. One in 10 used obviously youthful imagery, and nearly a third of all human images portrayed on the websites were people appearing to be 25 years of age or younger dressed in glitzy clothes, playing, smiling and laughing, giving the unmistakeable impression that poker was a glamourous activity for young people to engage in. Examples included Nasty Duck's 'Live Fast and Play Hard' and Rockem Poker's 'Because Your Life Rocks!' Three in every 10 of the sites used features such as newsletters, blogs, archives, press releases, tournament updates, information about future events around the world, news about successes of site teams, and discussion pages and chat rooms.

Almost all sites provided some means of allowing free practice or giving training of some kind. One in ten provided separate practice sites where players were tutored about the basics of poker games. Ninety percent offered 'free play programs' that allowed customers to play with free credit to get a feel for the games. Two-thirds included online dictionaries and glossaries of terms to tutor consumers in the idiosyncrasies of poker lingo – terms such as all-in, buy-in, check-raise, drawing hand, fixed limit, flop, kicker, nuts, position, river, stack. Half of the websites transmitted the message that poker was a game of skill, involving, for example, opportunities 'to outsmart, out bet and outplay everyone else on the table' (Party Poker), and 'Play better, play smarter, so never stop learning' (Aced). Several sites even claimed that poker was akin to a skilled sport.

Bonuses of different kinds were offered by nearly all, among them deposit bonuses, sign-up bonuses or welcome bonuses to new customers after they opened accounts – the kinds of incentives which the Nottingham Trent group found were so attractive to online players. Other frequent bonuses included reload, VIP, loyalty, reward, best-hand and royal-flush bonuses. Over 80% featured 'reward programs' – the longer you stay playing, the greater the cash reward. Party Poker, for example, offered 'Palladium Lounge Status' to their most valued and dedicated players to keep them playing often and longer. Over three-quarters offered 'affiliate programs' to effectively turn players into sales reps, persuading customers to partner with the gambling-provider company to sell the product to others for a fee or a share of takings. For example those who were induced to be affiliates of Manchester United Poker could earn a 25% revenue share from any player who was referred for the lifetime of their stay.

A dominant message throughout all of this was the continual emphasis on wins, winning and winners. As this chilling report puts it, 'Most [sites] . . . were overt in transmitting messages of economic gain, often displaying the size of prizes in large, bold dynamic symbols and words'. Winning was bolstered by the dramatisation of winners, both real and fictional. Nasty Duck for example included a chart showing the last 24 hours' biggest winners along with screen names and winning amounts on every page of the site. Most sites used message boards and screen displays to report significant winnings to other players, giving the impression that consumers were constantly winning and that another big win was coming up. Three-quarters of the sites appeared to promote the belief that poker afforded an alternative means to financial and social success. No iQ Poker, for example, said, 'Many players around the world make a living playing poker online'. Poker Joint told customers, 'Play Here . . . and be Famous!'

Three-quarters of sites published responsibility statements. All but one provided warnings about underage play, and a few gave advice to parents on how to prevent underage gambling. About half offered guidance to consumers on how to limit excessive gambling, mostly in the form of endorsing deposit limits. Everest Poker allowed customers to limit the time they played, and when the limit was reached they were disconnected from the game. But most of these responsibility statements were found to be 'parsimonious in style when compared to the fanfare surrounding promotional incentives, sponsorships and endorsements'.

Summing up, the Canadian group make the following comments. The sites portrayed gambling as eminently natural, taking risk as a pleasure, and losing as entirely acceptable. Possible social and economic harms got little mention. They speak of sites 'deploying presentation formats that skewed the likelihood of winning, the perceived number and value of prizes, and the number of winners to incite participation'. As many others have noted also (e.g. Konietzny, 2017), it was their view that the sites not only promoted 'dubious beliefs' regarding the probability of success but also exaggerated the importance of personal skill and playing talent.

Gambling promotion aligned with sport

It is the much increased alignment of gambling with sport that has given rise to particular alarm. The rise of 'in-play' or live-action sports betting, which provides multiple betting opportunities which come quick and fast during a sporting event, has increased the intensity of sports betting. Researchers, particularly in Australia, have explored the ways in which the marketing of sports betting has become embedded within sport and how it appeals to fan loyalty, with professional sporting teams linked to gambling products and celebrities such as professional tennis player Boris Becker, Australian international cricketer Shane Warne and World Cup-winning footballer Marcel Desailly used to help promote gambling; all with the effect of reinforcing the idea that gambling is a harmless leisure activity, fun and an easy way to win money (Gainsbury *et al.*, 2015; Hing *et al.*, 2015). Australian studies have exposed implicit messages about loyalty to favourite sports teams, masculinity and being able to demonstrate sporting knowledge implanted within gambling advertising, as well as how sports betting is becoming embedded within existing peer-group sporting rituals, a natural 'add on' to sport, a socially accepted normal activity among young male peer groups (Deans *et al.*, 2017; Thomas *et al.*, 2012).

In one study, 100 gamblers representing a diverse range of socio-demographic characteristics and forms of gambling were interviewed to obtain their perceptions of advertising (Thomas *et al.*, 2012). Many commented that if one was interested in professional sporting events, one was now *bombarded* with messages suggesting a bet. There now seemed to be an 'inextricable connection between sport and gambling'. It was now 'massive', 'full on', 'through the roof', 'in your face', 'aggressive', 'unnecessary', 'impossible to avoid'. One man in his 30s said:

> I was at the football on the weekend and there were people walking around the concourse handing out flyers for an internet gambling site. You see it on the scoreboards at halftime. If you're listening on the radio in the car, in the amount of commentary they'll put it in and just give a review of the odds while the game's going on.

And according to a woman in her 40s:

> It's just horrible. Every ten minutes, they'll have Sportsbet – Collingwood versus St Kilda. They've got the odds up all the time. St Kilda kicks a goal and up come the odds and "oh they changed a little bit". It's definitely to get people to think about, "Oh St Kilda is coming back, maybe I'll just go and, whip down and put ten bucks on them".

Blurring the boundaries between sport and gambling was thought to be giving legitimacy to the gambling industry: 'Having the commentary team crossing to the Betfair guy for the update maybe gives it a bit more of legitimacy than it should have. It's becoming part of the broadcast, rather than an ad'. The frequent offer of incentives was another recurring theme, variously described as 'whacking you with free gifts', 'wicked' and 'trying to suck you in'.

The perceived danger of the normalisation of gambling was a further main theme. Some commented that, whoever you were, the industry had a marketing strategy for you: 'They're working every angle. Depending on who you are, they're making it low key, they're making it sophisticated, they're making it attractive to women, they're making it whatever'. While the study was going on, there was considerable media commentary and debate in Australia about the role of 'live odds' promotions during sporting matches. Younger men especially felt that the amount of gambling advertising was sending a dangerous message about the social acceptability of gambling and its normalised relationship with being a sports fan, and men who had actively used online betting sites were concerned that the messages were aimed at those who were under the legal betting age.

Football is the biggest, wealthiest and most followed sport in Britain, so its potential role in gambling promotion and normalisation is huge. The top tier of

English football, the Premier League, which can boast many of the world's highest rated players, is one of the most lucrative television contracts, and matches are viewed around the globe. Official statistics such as those produced by Ofcom only take into account gambling adverts on commercial television, for example the well-known 'gangster' actor Ray Winstone's long running bet365 football adverts. But other ways gambling operators promote their products have been growing in importance. One of the most important is club sponsorship: as Welsh researcher Carwyn Jones (2017; Jones et al., 2019) puts it, the players become 'walking (or running) billboards'. Several high-profile European football teams, such as AC Milan and Real Madrid, have had sponsorship deals with online betting companies, and English teams have followed. In the 2004–5 English Premier League (EPL) season, only one club's shirts were sponsored by a gambling company (Middlesbrough – 888.com). By the 2016–17 season, half the EPL teams were sponsored by a gambling company, and by 2018–19 sponsorship had spread to the second tier of English football, with over half of England's top 44 clubs now with players carrying prominent advertisements for gambling. Other teams have gambling 'partners'. Liverpool FC, for example, had online bookmaker BetVictor as partner; their name appeared on training kits and on billboards at the ground. The close link with the game goes beyond relationships with individual clubs. The second, third and fourth tiers of English football are now the Sky Bet Championship, Sky Bet League 1 and Sky Bet League 2; the Scottish leagues are now the Ladbrokes leagues; and the Welsh premier league is sponsored by Dafabet.

The highest levels of gambling exposure are on commercial TV channels, but even on public sector broadcaster BBC, where direct advertising is not permitted, viewers are constantly exposed to gambling promotions. As Jones says, gambling adverts appear on 'every shirt logo, pitch side hoarding advert, logo on manager's training kit, logos on press conference and post-match interview "wall"'. The latter is the interview backdrop, covered in gambling companies' logos, which appears whenever the BBC covers a live FA Cup match or previews league matches or in programmes showing match highlights such as *Match of the Day* – a favourite programme of mine and millions of others. Views of company logos are replicated in magazines, posters, websites and social media platforms, and TV coverage can be seen live or later via iPlayer or equivalent. There is also a lot of indirect advertising, such as the regular references to gambling on popular commercial radio stations such as talkSport and in the Twitter feeds of high-profile players turned commentators such as Robbie Savage and Dietmar Hamann.

Although in Britain we have not yet been exposed to the Australian-style in-programme expert discussion of football betting odds, traditional in association with British horse racing, the exposure to football betting advertising is now massive and unavoidable. Carwyn Jones and colleagues analysed TV broadcasts from the EPL and the Euro 2016 Championships involving five matches and four separate broadcasters. Overall, they saw 1135 references to gambling covering 176 minutes of the total 1502 minutes (nearly 12%) of broadcast time. In some match broadcasts, this 'gambling visibility' figure was as high as 30%. At times, players' shirts, static boards and digital boards displaying gambling company logos were visible at the same time. The exposure to gambling promotion through watching televised football broadcasts, substantial when those analyses were being carried out, undoubtedly rose very considerably in the following few years. In recent editions of *Match of the Day*, I have seen promotions for online gambling companies bet365, 12Bet, 1xBet, Betway, W88, SportPesa, Fun88, Tempobet, MoPlay, ManBetX, M88 and others.

At the same time appeared logos for trading gambling companies eToro and FxPro. This has also been noted by Lopez-Gonzalez and Griffiths (2018b), who share the concern about the volume and penetration of sports betting marketing strategies exemplified by the 'gamblification' of English football, extending the discussion to include forex trading and fantasy-gaming sponsorships. They suggest that the symbolic linkage of sport and such newer gambling forms can become an issue of public health, especially affecting vulnerable groups such as minors and problem gamblers. Specifically, regarding 'trading', they refer to online trading and credit companies such as Unicredit and Plus500 starting to invest in sports competitions, 'a cross-fertilization of the sports and risk-taking industries'.

The same British–Spanish collaborative research group has analysed over 100 TV sports betting adverts from their two countries. They found that adverts targeted men almost exclusively, aligning betting with masculinity and male characteristics such as self-efficacy and control. 'In play' betting was depicted in nearly half, and the value of sports knowledge was emphasised. Free-money offers, humour and the use of celebrities – they cite evidence to suggest that the use of celebrities may lower the perceived risk of betting – enhanced the image of a controlled, fun activity. At the same time the betting depicted typically involved small stakes with large potential returns, implying low risk but the opportunity to win big. The overall impression given was that betting was high-control/low-risk behaviour, quite the opposite, it could be said, to the reality for many (Lopez-Gonzalez *et al.*, 2018a, 2018c).

Children and young people exposed to gambling advertising

Although football is not *aimed* at children, a significant proportion of the audience are children. For example, Ofcom (2013) statistics showed that over 1.3 million children (aged 4–15) watched England's UEFA Euro 2012 matches with France and Ukraine, and over 600,000 children watched the live UEFA Champions League final between Chelsea and Bayern Munich the same year. Twenty-five percent of the television audience for the English Premier League (EPL) were aged between 16 and 24 in 2016 (Jones, 2017), and 19% of the online audience were also in that age group. These younger viewers would have been exposed to all the gambling marketing during these broadcasts.

One important factor in these exposure levels is the loophole in the UK regulations that exempt sports betting adverts during televised sporting events. An exception was made to the general principle of a 9.00 pm watershed for gambling advertising to allow the advertising of sports betting around televised sporting events, most of which take place or at least begin before that time of the evening; however, such pre-watershed adverts must not include sign-up offers targeted at new customers. Carwyn Jones' (2017) analysis of EPL and Euro 2016 matches showed that exposure to both gambling advertisements and on digital advertising boards was significantly higher before 9.00 pm, when younger people are presumably more likely to be watching, ironic considering that children and young people are the ones the watershed is supposed to protect. A move has been made by some companies – in my view trivial and motivated by the fear of more significant reform – to ban adverts during, but not immediately before or after, live sports events beginning before 9.00 pm.

It is clear that gambling companies have not only been pushing the boundaries of what most people would judge considerate of children and young people's well-being, but also, in Britain's case at least, have been testing the limits of what regulations and recommendations permit. The British Code of Advertising Practice, produced by the Committee of Advertising Practice, has rules for the scheduling of gambling advertisements. It says that gambling adverts must not feature in programmes aimed specifically at children. In terms of gambling adverts themselves, they must not 'exploit the susceptibilities, aspirations, credulity, inexperience or lack of knowledge of under-18s or other vulnerable persons' or 'be likely to be of particular appeal to under-18's especially by reflecting or being associated with youth culture'. And the European Commission's Recommendations on Principles for the Protection of Consumers and Players of Online Gambling Services and for the Prevention of Minors from Gambling Online include advising against 'endorsements by well-known personalities or celebrities that suggest gambling contributes to social·success' (Lopez-Gonzalo & Griffiths, 2016).

Social media and gambling advertising

It is not only TV adverts which are to blame for the exposure of the new generation of children and young people to gambling promotion. As discussed in Chapter 2, the provision of gambling or gambling-like applications on social networking sites popular with children is another area which is leaving gambling regulators perplexed about what to do. But it is also the use of social media to *advertise* gambling which is of concern since it is young people who are the most likely to be active social media users. An Australian group (Gainsbury et al., 2015, p 3) was interested in the growing use by gambling operators of promotion on social media sites. Sites such as Facebook and Twitter, they said,

> allow companies to establish brand pages, which users can "like" or "follow" to receive updates and content. Any activity that users engage with on brand pages may then appear in the news feeds of their Facebook connections, either directly through users sharing content, or indirectly through paid promotions by companies to targeted individuals and their connections.

Paddy Power, for example, claimed in 2013 that they had over 1.7 million Facebook fans and Twitter followers. The Australian group studied 101 social media sites being operated in Australia by gambling providers, including 70 EGM venues, 13 casinos, 12 betting agencies and six lottery providers.

The study was conducted over four weeks in October 2013. Nearly 90% of the operators were using Facebook, with an average of 20,000 followers each. Half were using Twitter, with an average of 4,500 followers. The betting agencies were particularly heavy users of social media sites: the 11 such agencies which used Facebook had an average of just over 100,000 followers, and the 11 that used Twitter had 16,500. They found that operators were using social media to provide information about their brand products, types of bet and betting events and were promoting features to make betting easier, including easy payment options, e.g. Ladbrokes' 'Your Cash in a Flash . . . Withdraw your winnings from any ATM in Australia with our game-changing Ladbrokes Card', accompanied by a video. New users were encouraged by the emphasis on the ease of trialling a certain product, positioning it as a good introduction to the gambling products and advocating that novices 'give it a go'. The authors of this report claim that gambling was presented as 'glamorous, exciting, fun and action-packed'. Winning was emphasised by promoting jackpot and prize amounts, good odds of winning and recent large wins. Betting was encouraged by some messages which offered the provision of expert tips – bet365 was specifically mentioned in that context.

That Australian study found a number of ways in which gambling operators were encouraging people to engage with them, not only by directly referring to opportunities to gamble, but also by encouraging venue patronage, for example by promoting in-venue events, products and services, members' prize draws, boxing matches, food and beverage facilities, how venue proceeds were used to benefit community organisations, events for returning service people and so on. In comparison there was little evidence of responsible gambling information or messages. Only a small minority had any such information on their social media profiles, and when they did, it was not at all prominently displayed. There was occasional use of jokes and images that would certainly be against British Advertising Standards Authority rules; for example, one Facebook posting featured a photograph of a man, surrounded by children, thinking about being at the races with the caption 'Where would you rather be?'

They also found, as others have with gambling advertising generally, that gambling was aligned with sport in social media through linking betting with sporting events and on-field play and appealing to sports fans' team loyalties and interests, particularly when teams, competitions or stadia were sponsored by gambling companies. They refer to this as yet another way in which 'social media may provide a "soft" (i.e. unrestricted) entry that covertly acculturates youth to the processes and mentalities of an adult world of gambling'.

Another Australian concern about the long-term impact of gambling marketing on children and young people has been the club venues which provide activities that are utilised by families and children but which also provide gambling activities. One study, which examined marketing tactics for non-gambling and gambling activities in a sample of 65 registered clubs in New South Wales, found the clubs used various tactics to appeal to families and encourage parents to bring their children into venues. The authors hypothesised that marketing aimed at bringing children and families into gambling environments might play a role in shaping children's engagement in gambling later in life (Bestman *et al.*, 2016). Although gambling in private clubs is not such a prominent concern in Britain, it is the case that exposure of children and young people to gambling is not well controlled in such settings in Britain, and the same issue of child protection applies also to British pubs.

Conclusion

In this chapter I have highlighted studies that have drawn attention to the manipulative ways in which gambling is promoted. I have also tried to give a flavour of research which has exposed the forceful – some would say aggressive – and often misleading ways in which modern forms of gambling are advertised. Table 4.1 summarises some of the conclusions that can be drawn from the studies discussed in this chapter.

TABLE 4.1 Some of the main conclusions to be drawn from studies of how gambling is advertised

Gambling marketing has exploded in size	People feel 'bombarded' by gambling advertising which 'seems to be everywhere'
It uses a wide range of marketing strategies	Strategies include television, radio, newspapers and magazines, public adverts, direct mail, websites and social media
Winning is the central motive for gambling	People give various economic, personal and/or social reasons for gambling, but the hope of winning money is the personal reason most frequently given
Adverts highlight wins, winning and winners	Gambling advertising aims to enhance the perception of the chances of winning with the actual probability of winning rarely alluded to, giving a misleading impression of the likelihood of winning
The importance of skill is overemphasised	A device commonly employed is an exaggerated emphasis on the importance of personal skill, playing talent and being able to demonstrate sporting knowledge, with less emphasis on chance
Gambling is depicted as low risk/high control	Adverts typically depict betting as involving small stakes but with the opportunity for big wins; by comparison, the risks of gambling are underemphasised

(Continued)

TABLE 4.1 (Continued)

Online gambling is seductive	Online gambling is convenient, providing opportunity for 24-hour gambling; sites are often highly sophisticated, fast and easy to navigate, and players are attracted by various 'free bet' and bonus offers, expert tips or training or easy payment options
Gambling and sport are increasingly aligned	There has been growth in links between sporting teams and gambling products including sponsorship of clubs, competitions and stadia by gambling companies; betting, including live-action betting, has become embedded within sports including football, appealing to fans' interests and team loyalties
There is often an appeal to masculinity	Gambling advertising, especially sports betting advertising, often makes an appeal to masculinity, aligning betting with supposed male characteristics such as self-efficacy and control
Celebrities are used	Celebrities, especially sporting celebrities well known to children and young people, are used to help promote gambling
A significant proportion of the audience for gambling promotion are children	Sports betting advertising, particularly, tests the boundaries of official regulations and recommendations and of what most people would consider protective of children and young people's well-being

Among the most significant of these conclusions are two. One is the increased exposure of children and young people to gambling advertising, much aided by the infiltration of sport and social media. The other is how gambling is promoted in ways which not only use all the tricks of the advertising trade but which also try to give a false impression of what engaging in modern forms of gambling really entails – telling prospective customers it is a low-risk pastime, full of fun, with a good prospect of winning money. The reality of modern commercial gambling – an activity with a high likelihood of losing money and one that carries dangers of addiction, undermining other life activities and harmful to mental health – is concealed.

This bears on a central question, whether offering the prospect of monetary gain when play in total is bound to result in loss, which is necessarily true of all profit-making, commercial gambling, is essentially misleading. The following chapter delves more deeply into this question of whether modern gambling is fundamentally fraudulent.

5

IS MODERN GAMBLING FRAUDULENT? HOW PLAYERS ARE DECEIVED ABOUT THE CHANCES OF WINNING

The *Gambling Establishment* discourse that has underpinned gambling in the recent modern era claims that gambling – much of it now in the hands of large companies that operate internationally and which have had the power to bring governments on to their side – is an ordinary leisure commodity like any other. They had made much headway in persuading the rest of us to think of gambling that way and to accept it as largely harmless, indeed as something which brings economic, cultural and consumer benefit. In the face of mounting concern about the addictiveness of modern forms of gambling, the harm it gives rise to for individuals, families and communities and society as a whole, and the dangers it poses for children and young people, the Establishment discourse is now starting to be seen as bogus.

Part of the narrative about gambling which we were asked to accept was that people gamble purely for entertainment. But the principal personal motive for gambling – from which other motives follow, such as to experience excitement or to distract oneself from troubles – is to win money. And in the last chapter we saw how the way modern commercial gambling is promoted rests on that central motivation; it is 'wins, winning and winners' (Binde, 2009; Banks, 2014) that advertisements for gambling emphasise continually. By using a wide variety of tricks to appeal to the universal liking for money, the desire to gamble is as much created by those who provide and profit from it as it is desired by those who come to it.

This chapter will go further in asking questions about the very nature of modern forms of gambling themselves. Something we shall look at closely is the manner in which winnings are paid out in modern machine and online gambling. Such questions, although modern gambling presents them in a particularly stark form, are not in fact totally new. It is interesting to note that in the 1930s the highly regarded research organisation Mass Observation drew attention to the many smaller payouts which were an important feature of the weekly football pools then popular in Britain (Madge & Harrisson, 1939). By their reckoning, over a period of three years about 85% of those engaged in pools betting won something, however little. They recognised that this was a big part of what kept people engaged, a factor they thought was often ignored by opponents of the pools. As we shall see, they were quite correct in concluding that periodic small wins kept those who participated interested. The conclusion Mass Observation failed to draw, however, was that in the long run these apparent small wins were not really wins at all. For most, they were the means of keeping customers engaged while disguising the experience of overall loss.

The difference between then and now lies in the later development of more technologically sophisticated, more intense, more accessible, more vigorously promoted forms of gambling. The basic principle that engagement in gambling is maintained by what some have now clearly recognised as LDWs or 'losses disguised as wins' remains the same (Templeton *et al.*, 2014). Because of technological change and an Establishment that has been slow to see the dangers inherent in the way gambling has changed, it is becoming clear how false is the claim that modern gambling is an ordinary leisure commodity like any other, conforming to the rules of transparency and fairness that govern leisure commodities such as buying a ticket to watch a sports event or to go to the theatre.

How modern gambling machines are designed to deceive players

Addiction by design in Las Vegas

The most perceptive and comprehensive account of the dangers of innovations in gambling machine design has been given us by Natasha Schüll (2012), anthropologist and associate professor at the Massachusetts Institute of Technology. Her book, *Addiction by Design: Machine Gambling in Las Vegas*, has had quite an impact partly because of her thoroughness in researching the field and partly because she managed to get a lot of people to talk to her. The latter included people who had become addicted to playing machines, but also, unusually, she met a good number of industry people who spoke surprisingly openly. She made extended visits to Las Vegas between 1992 and 2007 and describes reading through years of machine manufacturers' trade magazines, press releases and annual reports, attending gambling industry expositions and conference panels and interviewing industry representatives.

Summing up the transformation of gambling machines brought about by technological innovation since the first machine was invented in the USA at the very end of the 19th century, Schüll (p 4) says:

> The one-armed bandits of yesteryear were mechanical contraptions involving coin slots, pull-handles, and spinning reels. Today's standard gambling

machines are complex devices assembled on a digital platform out of 1,200 or more individual parts. . . . Once a relatively straightforward operation in which players bet a set amount on the outcome of a single payline, today machine gambling begins with a choice among games whose permutations of odds, stakes size, and special effects are seemingly endless.

When it comes to electronic gambling machines (EGMs), there are a number of different types and differences between countries in the most popular types of machine. In some parts of the world, EGMs are still referred to as video slot machines or video lottery terminals. The word video is confusing to those who have a warm recollection of watching 'videos', most have nothing to do with lotteries, and the expression 'slot machine' or 'slots' is now well out of date. In fact there is so much about the terminology surrounding EGMs which only serves to add to the general public's confusion. Schüll carefully documents the technological transformations which have rendered modern EGMs quite unlike their predecessors of only a few decades ago. One particularly ominous development, first introduced by the company Bally in Australia in the late 1960s, was 'multiple pay lines', whereby a player could stake on more than one line of images (originally images of fruits, hence the expression 'fruit machines') at a time. This innovation was quickly taken up in the USA. In the early 1990s Aristocrat introduced the first nine-line, five coins machine, since when pay lines had increased to 50, 100 and, allowing winning combinations of symbols to line up in any direction or in no particular direction at all, up to several thousand 'lines'. The use of split screens took the multiplication effect still further. Bonus rounds or free spins added yet further complexity.

Natasha Schüll also describes 'video poker' as a further good example of the speed with which technology was being exploited in order to provide ever more diverse forms of, ever more enticing, machine gambling. Since the 1980s, many different versions of video poker had been invented, including multi-hand games such as *Triple Play Draw Poker*, which allowed players to play three hands at once and three times as many coins to bet with, accelerating play and increasing the frequency of payouts. They were overtaken later by *Five Play, Ten Play*, even up to *Hundred Play Poker* and *Spin Poker* which combined multiple hands of video poker with the multiple pay lines of Australian-style pokie machines. Such technological EGM developments continue unabated. In Britain, as described in Chapter 1, it was the EGMs which provided electronic casino-type games via machine – the Fixed Odds Betting Terminals, so called – which took advantage of the technological possibilities and made EGMs so much quicker and greedier.

Schüll was quite clear about the role played by the very design of modern gambling machines. All the interviews she carried out, with both gamblers and industry reps, convinced her that the machines were designed – and deliberately so – in order to induce and reinforce personal motivation. To her, it was abundantly obvious that the need to gamble, and to carry on gambling, was as much created as pre-existing. An important part of her thesis was that playing gambling machines provides 'a reliable mechanism for securing a zone of insulation . . . hold[ing] worldly contingencies in a kind of abeyance, granting . . . an otherwise elusive zone of certainty.' One person she spoke to said, 'You're in a trance, you're on autopilot'; another said, 'I go into a tunnel vision where I actually do not hear or see anything around me . . . the only thing that exists is the screen'. Others have used the expression 'dark flow' – indexed by agreement with such statements as, 'I forgot everything around me', 'I lost track of time', 'I was deeply concentrated in the game' and 'I lost connection with the outside world' – to refer to the same phenomenon (Dixon et al., 2018a).

Although the industry claims that what players want is entertainment or 'fun', Schüll found industry representatives who recognised something different. For example, Gardner Grout of Silicon Gaming said,

> What we didn't get at the beginning is that people don't really want to be entertained. *Our best customers are not interested in entertainment* – they want to be totally absorbed, they want to get into a rhythm.

Bally's Bruce Rowe said,

> Innovation should not stifle the main purpose of our business, which is machine revenue. We can drive down revenue by putting features in front of players that divert them from their primary goal – which is to play the machine. *We're not in the entertainment business; this is still gambling* (pp 168, 170, original emphases).

Canadian research shows how volatility disguises the operator's advantage

Some of the best work on the intricacies of modern machine gambling, and by extension modern commercial gambling in general, has come from Canadian researchers. Most modern commercial forms of gambling have a complicated multi-level prize structure consisting of some combination of small, medium and jackpot prizes and, in the case of large lotteries, a minute possibility of an enormous prize. In the case of much sports betting, as well as some casino games such as roulette, the player can pre-select a preferred prize option, choosing a more likely outcome at small odds or a less likely outcome at longer odds. Technological advances, including multi-line and multi-hand games, bonus rounds of various kinds, and linked machines, made even greater variation possible.

Because of the multi-level prize structure of EGMs there is a high degree of what is termed 'volatility' in the potential outcome from bet to bet. Volatility is usually measured as the amount of variation in outcome after 10,000 spins or bets. Simple even-money games such as baccarat have a very low level of volatility, and lotteries, with their enormous jackpots, a very high level. Gambling machines lie somewhere in between but vary a great deal depending upon their prize structure.

Those that offer a lot of small prizes but also large jackpots have a higher volatility than those that only offer small or medium-sized prizes.

One highly significant effect of volatility of outcome when playing EGMs is that it makes it difficult for players to judge how fair the game is. This can be shown by writing a computer programme that simulates the likely outcomes of playing an EGM for varying lengths of time, which is exactly what Ontario researcher Nigel Turner (2011) did and reported in an article in the *Journal of Gambling Studies*. He ran multiple simulations of playing three different types of EGM. One gave mostly small prizes, a second mostly gave medium prizes, and the third, more volatile machine gave small prizes but with a very large jackpot. He set the simulations to bet at a rate of 600 times an hour; in other words one spin every six seconds, which he says is a fairly conservative figure for modern EGMs – itself an extraordinary figure giving us some indication of what a strange form of entertainment this is! The house advantage was set at 7.5%, which is fairly average.

Under those conditions he was able to show that on the less volatile machines it would take about 70 hours of play before the number of winners dropped to less than a tenth of one percent, although it would take ten times that period of play before the chances of ending up on the winning side dropped to that level on the more volatile machine. This just shows the obvious fact that if you keep on playing such machines for long enough your chances of ending up a winner are as near to zero as makes no difference. However, what this exercise in simulation also showed very clearly is why during a relatively short period of play it is so difficult to appreciate how it is that the chances of ending up a winner are decreasing all the time, sooner or later decreasing to virtually nothing. This inexorable downward trend is, as Turner put it, 'masked by the number of wins'. All the simulated 'players' who persisted continued to win small amounts from time to time – just as Mass Observation noted for the football polls years ago. There were some who won a comparatively large amount, particularly when volatility was high, although even they would give it back to the machine if they persisted in playing.

Turner went on to quantify the difficulty players might have in appreciating the long-term outcomes of play by calculating a statistic known as the 'effect size' (for those interested in the statistics, this was the ratio of the average expected loss to the standard deviation of expected loss after a particular interval of play). He calculated that after an hour's play on any of these machines the effect size is small and therefore difficult to detect. In order for the effect to become a large and therefore easily detectable one, it would be necessary to make between 2,400 and 6,000 spins on the relatively low-volatility machines and as many as 30,000 spins on the high-volatility one.

His not unreasonable conclusion was that commercial EGMs are designed 'to maximize the number of short term winners and minimize the number of long term winners'. For any short length of play – for example less than 2,400 spins – it is difficult for a player to appreciate the house advantage. This provides part of the answer to the puzzle of why people are not more aware that the machine is fixed in such a way that their chances of winning if they keep on playing are slender. As Turner (2011, pp 19–20) put it:

> They are essentially lost in the forest of wins caused by the volatility of the game, and this makes it hard to appreciate the long term losses. . . . The high volatility of multilevel prize games hides the house edge so that the player cannot tell during any short period of play that the game has a built in advantage for the casino. . . . In general the gambling industry is risk averse and does not gamble. . . . Prize structures selected for EGMs enhance player appeal by providing the players with many frequent prizes to keep the player interested, mixed in with less frequent larger prizes that make a miraculous recovery possible.

Why information about payback percentage is mostly misleading and irrelevant

From the same part of the world, Kevin Harrigan and Mike Dixon (2009) studied a different but closely related feature, namely the payback percentages offered by different machines. They used the Canadian Freedom of Information and Protection of Privacy Act to obtain the Probability Accounting Report (PAR) sheets for slot machines approved in Ontario. Otherwise known as 'paytable and reel strip sheets', these provide details of such things as the configuration of a game's reels, pay combinations, payback percentages, hit frequency and volatility index. They are normally a matter of commercial secrecy. Harrigan and Dixon were able to show how difficult it must be for most players to distinguish machines with very different payback percentages. In practice the payback percentage of machines in Ontario varied widely, typically from a low of 85% to a high of 98%, or, to put it a different way, the operator's edge or advantage varied from 15% to 2%. Regulations about this vary from country to country and often from state to state or province to province. In Britain, for example, operators are obliged to display the payback percentage, or return to player (RTP) as it is called, but it has been shown that this is not widely understood (Collins, 2014), and in any case it can be highly misleading, as we shall see.

These researchers studied a type of machine, popular in Ontario at the time, called *Lucky Larry's Lobstermania*. They noted that there were multiple 'help' screens available on the machine that explained how to play the game, and lists of all winning combinations and their associated winning amounts were made available but *not* the odds of winning each prize *nor* the machine's payback percentage. Simply from studying the PAR sheets they were able to draw some interesting conclusions. For example, the machine displayed five reels with between 46 and 50 symbols per reel, yielding a staggering just over 250 million possible outcomes. The possibility of a jackpot was advertised but on average would be won just once in over eight million spins.

Their computer simulations gave, as might be expected, very different results from the two types of machine. Starting with $100, spinning every six seconds, a player on the low-payback machine could expect on average to play for half an hour before the money was exhausted, spinning 178 times and winning something on 56 of those spins. Playing the high-payback version, on the other hand, a player might expect to be able to carry on playing for an average of just over two hours and twenty minutes, spinning 1,333 times and winning something on 435 of those spins. The jackpot remained elusive; even on the high-payback machine there remained only a one in 400 chance of making it. More likely were invitations to enter an optional extra 'bonus mode'.

The importance of skewed distributions of wins

But those are arithmetic averages. Crucially, they give a very distorted impression of the experience of *the average gambler* playing such machines. This is because, due to the random schedule according to which wins occur on a minority of spins and not on others and according to which different denominations of wins are assigned, the amounts that players win on gambling machines are distributed in a highly skewed way. This idea of a highly skewed distribution of wins is basic for understanding the deception involved in machine gambling and for appreciating the 'price' that the large majority of gamblers are paying. In fact, it is basic for understanding the deception involved in all modern forms of high intensity – continuous, fast, volatile – commercial gambling. But it may be a bit tricky to understand. In plain terms, what it means is that the larger number of players, if they win at all, win relatively small amounts, while smaller and yet smaller pro-portions of players win larger and yet larger amounts. In other words, only a small minority of players win a lot, and their winnings contribute disproportionately to the average payback. This is why, even in jurisdictions where it is a requirement to provide payback percentage or return-to-player information, this is misleading. A return-to-player percentage of 90% might, quite incorrectly, be interpreted as meaning that there is a 90% chance of being a winner. It masks the fact that the majority of players will lose.

Using medians as a better indication of the experience of the average player, Harrigan and Dixon were able to clearly show that the experience for most players would be very little different depending on whether a low-payback or high-payback version of the machine was being played. In either case, the 'average' player (i.e. the median or middle of the range player) would be able to play for only about a quarter of an hour before money was exhausted, making only slightly more spins on the high-payback machine (101 versus 81) and winning only very slightly more often (on 32 versus 26 spins). Furthermore, the median player would never in that time experience the bonus mode, let alone the jackpot.

Probably the most interesting figures of all emerging from this simulation exer-cise were the payback percentages that the median players could expect. Instead of the average percentages (that is, the real mathematical averages) of 85% and

98% – which were confirmed by the results of the simulations – the median values were 66.5% for the low-payback machine and not much better at 72.9% for the high-payback machine. It appears, therefore, that not only were the advertised payback percentages misleadingly high, but also the difference between machines was almost completely irrelevant for most players!

This astute Canadian duo went further, suggesting that the higher the payback advertised percentage, the more dangerous is the activity of playing! In countries where the RTP is advertised openly, players are likely to be attracted to machines with apparently higher RTP and may not realise that in the process they are running an even greater risk of developing a problem. That is because there would be more 'big winners' on the higher payback machine. For example, on the low-payback machine there would be only five players out of 1,000 who at some stage would have reached a peak balance of more than $1,000, but on the high-payback machine there would be 54 of them. It was these big winners in the tail of the highly skewed distribution of winnings who accounted for the big differences in the arithmetic average, leaving everyone else, whichever version of the machine they were playing, running out of their money relatively quickly and having comparatively very few experiences of winning.

There is consensus that EGMs are a particularly addictive form of gambling (e.g. MacLaren, 2015; Orford et al., 2013; Sulkunen et al., 2019), and having a 'big win' is something that people with gambling problems very frequently describe having experienced early on in their gambling careers (e.g. Custer & Milt, 1985). Furthermore, those who are big winners are also having the experience of being able to bet for a longer period of time, having many more spins and more experiences of winning, all of which is likely to lead to stronger habit learning and therefore be particularly dangerous. So, it seems that information about payback percentage or return to player is not only misleading but, for most players, irrelevant. If these researchers' conclusions are right, higher payback machines are even more addictive than those which on average return a lower percentage to players.

Online sports gamblers are also being deceived about the odds of winning

That same deceptive claim, that their customers are being given the opportunity to win money when in fact nearly all are losing nearly all the time, is equally true of those who provide gambling online. Remember from the last chapter how forcefully online gambling providers sell the prospect of winning money. In 2007, a team from Harvard Medical School published what may well have been, as they claimed, 'the first ever analysis of real-time betting behavior of Internet sport gamblers' (LaBrie et al., 2007). It involved a single online sports gambling service provider, bwin. The latter made available to the research team a complete eight months record of the sports betting activity with their service of all, just over 40,000, sports bettors from 85 countries, mostly in Europe, who opened an account with the company during the whole of a single month. In total, over the next eight months, they placed 5.3 million outcome bets and 2.5 million live-action bets. On average they placed four bets a day. Those who bet on outcomes – nearly everyone in the sample – wagered in total an average of €729 and made an average net loss of €97. Those who made live-action bets at any time – about 60% of the sample – wagered on them a total of €1,319 each and lost €85 on average. However, as we have noted above, when it comes to gambling data, averages are very misleading. That is because, as the Harvard group pointed out, most of their measures were heavily skewed. They gained further insight into this by examining the data from three extreme and overlapping subgroups: the 1% who ran up the heaviest net losses, the 1% who wagered the most in total and the 1% who placed the largest number of bets. The summary figures for their betting are staggering. Amongst outcome bettors, the last of those groups bet no less than 37 times a day and placed almost 3,500 bets on average during the six to seven months in which they were active. The high total-wagered group wagered an average of nearly €23,000, and the extreme net-loss group lost an average of nearly €3,500!

The other important point which the authors note, which I commented on earlier in the context of machine gambling, is that the percentage return to player (RTP) depends on how it is calculated. If it is calculated by dividing the total sum of losses – which was just under €4 million in the case of outcome betting – by the total amount of money wagered – nearly €30 million – the percentage loss appears to be 13%, or in other terms an RTP of 87%. The equivalent figures for live-action betting appeared even better for players at 6% for percentage loss and hence an RTP of 94%. These figures, the authors say, are in agreement with the target returns expected by the operator bwin. However, if percent losses are calculated separately for each individual player and then averaged, the average percent lost turns out to be much greater: 32% in the case of outcome bets and 23% for live-action bets, making it appear that the average percentage RTP is much less generous, at 68% and 77%. The total amount wagered by individuals and their net loss percentages were negatively correlated. In other words, small bettors, who bet less and therefore contributed less to the calculation of overall loss percentage, actually lost a higher percentage of everything they bet. The bigger bettors won more often and their loss percentage was therefore on average lower. But of course they lost more in total. It can therefore be said that this internet gambling provider was making its money from a combination of lots of small bettors who tend to lose a relatively large proportion of the small amounts they bet and a smaller number of large bettors who lose a lot in absolute terms although not in relation to the very large amounts which they wager. But the important point is that online sports bettors, like players of modern gambling machines, are being deceived about the real odds of winning (see Figure 5.1).

Just as interesting as the results of this paper is how the authors interpreted their results in a way that might be seen as favourable to the online gambling-providing industry. The Harvard group has become somewhat notorious for receiving money from the industry and has been accused of showing bias towards favouring interpretations that serve industry interests (Adams, 2016; Kindt, 2012). In the

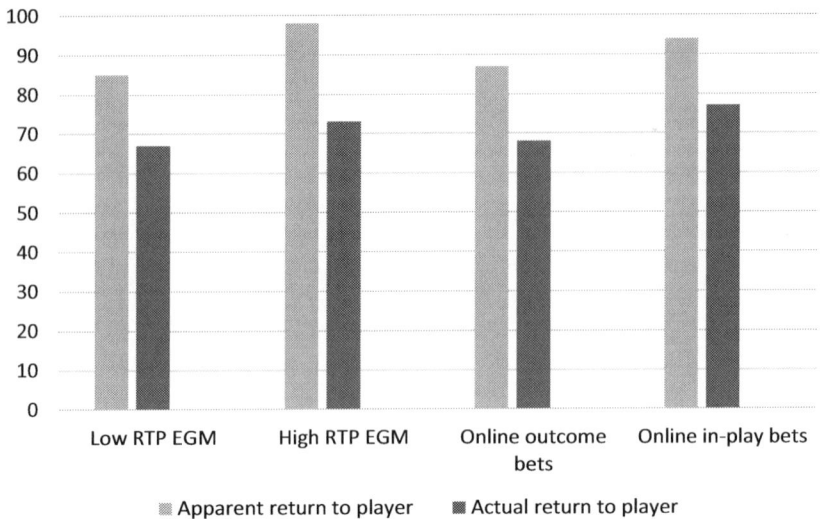

FIGURE 5.1 Examples of apparent and actual percent return to player (RTP) for EGM and online sports betting (EGMs with relatively low and high RTP, Harrigan & Dixon, 2010; Online outcome and in-play betting, LaBrie *et al.*, 2007)

discussion of their findings, they emphasised the relatively moderate gambling activity of most subscribers, saying, 'The findings reported here do not support the speculation that Internet gambling has an inherent propensity to encourage excessive gambling among a large proportion of players'. Rather than considering the complete distribution of gambling from small to large scale, they focus on 'extreme' groups constituting only 1% of the sample. They claim that the results indicate 'a clear discontinuity' between the 1% groups and the remainder of the sample although they present no convincing evidence of such discontinuity. This is another case of the all too common misinterpretation of skewed distribution curves. It is also notable that although the authors focus on these extreme 1% groups, when discussing their findings they do not draw attention to the very large amounts of money which those groups lost gambling online during a period of just a few months. And even those figures, colossal though they are, are likely to be underestimates since some will have been betting at the same time with other providers. We shall see more evidence of bias in the interpretation of research in Chapter 8.

Losses disguised as wins: a concept which throws light on the deceptiveness of modern commercial gambling of any type

One of the important features of many modern machines which the simulations described earlier were not able to examine is the option available to play on more than one line at a time. The same group of Canadian researchers went on to expose an important effect of that option (Templeton *et al.*, 2014). When it is available, as it is on machines in Australia and Canada for example, it has been shown a number of times that players do indeed prefer to bet on more than one line simultaneously. Some have speculated that this may partly be due to the regret that a player might experience if it is found that a win could have been achieved if other lines had been played. The increased possibility of large wins and bonus features may be an additional attraction of playing several lines at a time.

What this group of researchers pinpointed was the likelihood that when players play on several lines at a time, they may have the impression that they have won on a particular spin when in fact they have lost. This is even more likely because every win on a single line is celebrated – for example with the playing of a celebratory song and the lighting up of winning symbols – even though the other lines which a player bet on are losses on that spin (it is known that accompanying sounds and music effects increase player arousal: Spenwyn *et al.*, 2010). For example, if $.10 is bet on each of ten lines, a win of $.20 on one of those lines will be celebrated as a win, although overall on that spin the player has lost $.80. These researchers referred to such outcomes as 'losses disguised as wins' or LDWs, a concept which goes a long way to throwing light on the deceptiveness of modern commercial gambling of any type.

Previous research had indicated that players tend to overestimate the amount they are winning because they misinterpret LDWs as wins. The Canadians confirmed that finding and went further, using a number of ingenious methods to show that players experience LDWs differently than real losses, displaying a higher level of arousal following LDWs than following real losses. For example, after LDWs, players paused longer before the next spin (as they did after a real win: a phenomenon known in behavioural psychology as the 'post-reinforcement pause') and pressed the spin button harder. In these respects, LDWs are experienced more like real wins.

A Norwegian study confirmed the LDW effect in a real-world setting. It examined the records of over 8,000 individuals who made over two million bets in the course of one day on EGMs operated by the Norwegian state monopoly Norsk Tipping. The crucial measure here was whether players continued to bet in the same session. As expected from the Canadian work, although players were most likely to carry on gambling after an actual win, they were more likely to carry on playing after a loss that was disguised as a win than after a real loss (Leino *et al.*, 2016).

This idea of LDWs is highly significant. It not only helps us understand how modern multi-line EGMs motivate continued gambling by deceiving players into thinking that they are winning when they are actually losing but also gives us an important insight into how all gambling works. The LDW effect was identified in the context of multi-line EGM gambling where it is fairly obvious when pointed out – although it took the Canadian research programme to do so – that an LDW, however much razzmatazz is associated with it, is really a loss. But so too are the wins, mostly small, that a player experiences in the course of a session of playing an EGM that ends, as most do, with an overall loss. So too are the online betting wins that an online gambler experiences in the course of several weeks or months of betting before finally realising that in total the experience has been one of loss. The wins along the way can reasonably be thought of as losses disguised as wins. Only when the totality of the experience across multiple lines, spins and bets across hours, weeks or months is appreciated, does this become clear.

Other ways of seducing gamblers into spending more: near misses, complex and in-play bets, and the illusion of skill and control

The LDW concept is a relative newcomer in gambling studies. Another, long-recognised way of encouraging an over-inflated perception of the likelihood of winning is to arrange that players experience a greater than chance frequency of *near misses*. B F Skinner, the father of behavioural psychology, made the observation in the 1950s that almost winning encouraged machine players to keep going, costing the provider nothing in the process. By chance there are bound to be many times when gamblers have the experience of almost winning, but not quite. Illogical though it mostly is, this is bound to encourage further attempts to win. What is not inevitable, however, but which undoubtedly happens (Schüll, 2012), is when the design of the game, machine or operation deliberately enhances the chances of experiencing near misses.

One of the most dangerous features of some forms of gambling, but not all, is the way they allow repetitive or continuous gambling. In-play betting is a specially significant development in that respect. As Lopez-Gonzalez and Griffiths (2016) wrote, it has 'subverted the traditional episodic nature of sports betting . . . betting as a discontinuous form of gambling has given way to a continuous form of gambling'. In-play betting might, they suggest, be on its way to becoming the leading form of sports betting in Europe. They cited the Betfair annual report for 2015 as suggesting that the number of matches allowing in-play betting might have increased by over 100% between 2014 and 2015, and they further cited a 2015 report by the Spanish gambling regulator that 74% of money bet online on sports in Spain came from in-play betting. New developments included video game-like environments, fantasy sports games and in-play mini-games. As they commented, 'the technological evolution of the gambling industry seems unrelenting'.

Another long-recognised source of deception is the deliberate encouragement of an erroneous perception of skill and agency on the gambler's part (Langer & Roth, 1975). For example, allowing a player to select the number of lines played on a multi-line EGM appears to give the player some control over the game, encouraging the 'illusion of control' and the false sense that some skill is involved. In Britain some years ago we got used to new EGM features such as 'hold' and 'nudge' buttons and 'trails' of a number of steps which had to be completed in order to win a jackpot. Such features also encourage the feeling that the player has some control over the outcome, fostering the illusion that there was some skill involved.

Despite appearances, pressing a hold or stop button makes no difference to the outcome, which is wholly determined by a random number generator as soon as the player presses the spin button. If asked, most players will say they are not fooled by this (but not all: Dixon *et al.*, 2018b, found that 14% of their participants had erroneous cognitions about the stop button). But, in yet another study from the Canadian group, it was shown that a stop button does have an effect on arousal. Gamblers recruited from a casino in Ontario played two versions of a slot machine simulator: one with a stop button and one without. They assessed players' arousal following wins, losses and near misses by using their measures of skin conductance response (SCR), pressure on the spin button and post-reinforcement pauses. As predicted, players depressed the spin button harder, and had larger SCRs, whatever the outcome – win, loss or near miss – when using the stop button. They also paused longer following near misses when there was a stop button (Dixon *et al.*, 2018b).

Another way betting companies have found to deceive gamblers into thinking they have more control than they actually do have is to offer complex rather than simple bets; for example, that a football team will not just win but win by a three-goal margin, or that a particular player will be the one to score a goal, or, more complex still, that there will also be more than a certain number of corner kicks in the match. The teams and players named are usually very well-known and popular and the bets, though complex, appear credible to those who follow the sport closely. Of course, the outcomes of these bets, though they appear highly credible, are in reality more unlikely than they appear to be, with the result that the payout is significantly lower than for simpler bets (Newall, 2015, 2017). In the Sheffield Hallam analysis of online gambling promotions (see Chapter 4), some promotors were even found to be suggesting, on the contrary, that multiple bets actually *increased* the probability of winning. For example:

> The great thing about multiple betting is your stake stays the same – but your chances of winning big money multiply as the odds just keep getting bigger.
>
> Andrew from London kicked off the new season on the right foot with an easy win! He placed a £10 accumulator on 10 teams, mixing up the likes of Man Utd, Sheff Utd, Torquay, Sussex and St Helens in the football, cricket & rugby. After watching them all come in, Andrew collected a cool £1278.71!
>
> (Banks, 2014, pp 56–57)

The importance of gambling venues

I have been concentrating in this chapter on some of the abstruse and mystifying ways in which modern forms of gambling, because of the very structure of the way they are designed, deceive players about their real chances of winning – or of losing, which would be the more apt way of putting it. But of course the seductiveness, and for many the addictiveness, of modern gambling lies in more than just the design of the machines themselves or the structure of odds and payouts. It lies also in the locations and designs of the settings in which gambling is offered – a topic which in itself deserves more attention than I can give it here.

The importance of setting is abundantly clear in the case of casino design. Natasha Schüll (2012) quotes from a 1972 book by architects Venturi and colleagues, *Learning from Las Vegas*: 'The combination of darkness and enclosure of the gambling room and its subspaces makes for privacy, protection, concentration and control. . . . One loses track of where one is and when it is'. Of the casinos started by casino tycoon Steve Wynn, she says,

> Although Wynn has downplayed the role of such strategy in the design of his own casinos . . . in fact each of his properties has been a fastidiously planned affair from conception to finish, from wall treatments to ambient soundtrack.

She also quotes extensively from a 2000 book, *Designing Casinos to Dominate the Competition* (Friedman, 2000), which talks about designing casinos to encourage gamblers' entry into 'secluded, private playing worlds. . . [in] small alcoves, recesses, and corners'. Deliberate design features include what some industry consultants have called 'casino atmospherics' which includes controlling temperature, light, colour, sound and even aroma. Distractions such as music that is too loud or varied are avoided in case they should 'restore[s] . . . your cognitive state to where you can make rational decisions', as one analyst of casino design had noted.

How easily accessible gambling is was the focus of a study from Melbourne which used focus groups and interviews with gamblers to look at two types of accessibility: what they termed *geo-temporal* accessibility and *social and personal* accessibility (Marshall & Baker, 2001). By the former was meant such things as whether gambling venues were close to home and open for long hours every day, whether a number of different opportunities to gamble were available at any given venue (for example a casino offering several floors dedicated to different forms of gambling, the greater variety of games offered online, or a modern EGM offering a choice of games and formats), or whether people passed gambling venues *en route* to work, at their local shopping centres and in social or community hubs. As one woman participant said,

> I go to the supermarket and I feel tired and I feel drained just fighting the urge to go [to gamble] and I get up near the supermarket to actually buy food and right across the road will be a pokie venue.

Some venues used courtesy buses to provide door-to-door transportation, which could dramatically increase perception of accessibility particularly for those without private transport or with physical disabilities.

Included in the category of social and personal accessibility were such things as whether a gambling venue is seen to be attractive and non-threatening, whether membership and a certain code of dress are required as conditions of entry, whether the initial outlay required is low or high, and whether products are thought to be easy to use or seen as requiring skill – casino card games such as Texas hold 'em poker, for example, might be complicated to the uninitiated, whereas purchasing a raffle ticket is a simple task. Social accessibility turned out to be a surprisingly important theme, and there were several aspects to it. One aspect was it being a social place: 'a place where you can sit down and chill out and have a quiet beer, a little dabble on the pokies, just pass a couple of hours'. Another aspect was that a venue could be an accessible retreat where you could 'get lost in this virtual world'; 'All your cares seem to stay outside the door . . . you just dump them for a while'. Financial accessibility was important to some: 'What ATMs have they got there? How easy is it to get money if I have to go out for money? . . . all those things are part of your decision of how quick can I gamble'.

Another aspect, particularly important for women, was venue safety. As one woman in the Melbourne study said: 'A woman by herself can go nowadays . . . it is very safe, they have security there, they have door men, and if you (are) there late at night they escort you right up to the car'. It has been suggested that venue safety has been an important factor in what many have seen as the feminisation of gambling in the modern era, with domestic or otherwise female-friendly settings such as comfortable pokie venues in Australia, ordinary, unthreatening retail outlets for purchasing lottery tickets, and now at-home online gambling (Bowden-Jones & Prever, 2017), as opposed to male environments such as competitive poker or British betting shops. In Britain and elsewhere, bingo, regularly found in surveys to be the one form of gambling more favoured by women than men, has served as a woman-friendly setting for decades. In fact, based on survey data going back to the late 1940s, Heather Wardle (2017) makes a convincing case for saying that, if there has been a recent feminisation of British gambling, it would be more appropriate to call it a re-feminisation since there is evidence, from a 1951 survey particularly, that women were much more engaged in horse race and football pools betting than they were 60 years later. The change she suggests is likely due to the changed environment in which betting took place once it was legalised – no longer were betting slips collected from one's home but now in austere, male-dominated betting shops.

Online gambling, available 24/7 without the need to enter any special venue, now offers almost limitless space-time accessibility. Furthermore, as participants in the English Nottingham Trent study (McCormack & Griffiths, 2012, see Chapter 4) told researchers, the anonymity offered by internet gambling, and the avoidance of feelings of intimidation and the risk of 'losing face' for those who do not know the rules or are inexperienced, are other attractions. As Fran – not her real name – said, 'if you're gambling in a bookies, people are going to notice . . . whereas Internet gambling is hidden away, there's only you and your computer'.

Conclusion: gamblers are now being deliberately misled about the chances of winning

We saw in the previous chapter how an emphasis on winning is pervasive in the promotion of modern gambling despite the *Gambling Establishment's* emphasis on gambling as simply entertainment. In this chapter we have seen how modern EGMs and online sports betting are structured in such a way that gamblers are continually being misled about their chances of winning. Does this amount to manipulation? Does it mean that much of what is now offered as gambling is inherently fraudulent? Normal principles of consumer protection would require that consumers of gambling products should be given adequate price information in the form of the real odds of winning. This appears not to be happening. There may be an indication of the theoretical payout percentage or 'return to player' (RTP), but that is deceptive because it seriously underestimates the real operator advantage or 'house edge'.

Throughout her book *Addiction by Design*, Natasha Schüll (2012) raises the question of the extent to which designers, marketers and managers of gambling machines – and the same applies to online sports and other forms of modern gambling – should be held accountable. I believe she is right to conclude that 'Industry designers actively martial technology to delude gamblers', that there is an 'information asymmetry' between gambling operator and customer, and that it is the operator that has 'the upper hand'.

There has probably always been this element of deception in gambling, but a combination of the exploitation of digital technology and the encouragement of liberalising governments has made it now more malign and treacherous than it has ever been. Remember what Mass Observation said about people doing the football pools in the 1930s – the chances of a really big win were slight but most had experiences of small wins which kept them motivated. So is that what gambling is all about? Is that why we do it? We are really losing, but we keep on having experiences that make us think we are really winning. We are being deceived. Or are we? Don't all gamblers know the score? They know they are very likely to lose over a period of time and that small wins along the way, enjoyable though they are, do not alter that fact. What the Canadian machine research seems to show, however, is that we are easily deceived at some level of consciousness and, furthermore, that modern machines are purposely designed to take advantage of that. The same basic process of deception was going on years ago when British football pools companies delivered their coupons to people's homes – a service that was finally withdrawn in the 1950s – and, after carefully filling them in, our grandparents waited until the following Saturday to find out if they had won anything. What has changed is not the basic dynamics of the process, nor perhaps the fundamental deception behind it, but rather the speed and intensity involved and the use made of advanced technology. If persuading our forebears to carry on betting on the weekend football was not a con trick, enticing people to continue putting money into a modern gambling machine certainly is.

In the hands of inventive modern gambling entrepreneurs, forms of gambling are now much more diverse, and many of them are greatly more sophisticated than they were in the days when the rights and wrongs of football pools gambling were being debated. The word 'sophisticated' can be taken in different ways. To those who think that modern developments have simply added to entertainment value, and hence to consumer surplus in economists' language, it means something positive. But it means something more sinister to those who believe in fairness and to those who have been entrapped by these new developments. In the following chapter we turn to consider those who have suffered the most from the deceptiveness of modern gambling, who have experienced its power and dangerousness at closest quarters – those who become addicted to it.

6

UNDERSTANDING GAMBLING ADDICTION

Bringing personal experience and theory together

At the heart of the view of commercialised gambling which the industry and the rest of the *Gambling Establishment* has so keenly wanted us to accept is the idea that modern gambling products are essentially safe. Only a minority of people, sometimes dishonestly referred to as a 'tiny' minority, can't or won't use them safely, so the argument runs, and there is something wrong with many such people irrespective of their gambling. The fault they say lies not in the product but in the person. I now want to challenge that belief head on. In this chapter we shall hear from people who know from their own experience how dangerous gambling can be. But first let me begin by talking about the peculiar phenomenon of self-exclusion.

The strange case of self-exclusion and what it says about modern gambling

Self-exclusion may seem like an odd place to begin a chapter on gambling addiction. But it occupies a prominent role in debates about modern gambling. There are two reasons for that. The first is simply the existence of a broad consensus that it is one of the ways of trying to combat the harms associated with gambling. A good example is the self-exclusion system operating in the Swiss canton of Ticino, close to the Italian border (Sani & Zumwald, 2017), where three of Switzerland's 21 casinos are situated. Every customer has the right to request exclusion, either at the casino during a visit or by letter, and is then required to complete a form including socio-demographic information, the reason for the exclusion request, financial information, gambling behaviour and a problem gambling screening questionnaire. Exclusion is for at least one year, and further extensions can then be requested, leading to an hour-long interview. All Swiss casinos are networked so that the exclusion agreement applies across the country.

Many other jurisdictions provide programmes to allow gamblers to arrange to be excluded from gambling venues, thereby seeking to prevent or limit gambling-related harm. The first formal self-exclusion programme is thought to have been in Manitoba, Canada, in 1989 when the province's first permanent casino was established. Since then similar programmes have been initiated in other Canadian provinces, several US states, New Zealand, Australia and several European and Asian countries (Gainsbury *et al.*, 2014). Periods of self-exclusion vary. The Swedish *Spelpaus* system, for example, allows options varying from an initial one month up to 12 months (iGB Affiliate, 2019). Systems in other countries allow longer periods, up to five years in some cases.

Self-exclusion is particularly well developed in Australia and New Zealand and also in some European countries, at least for casino gambling. For example, almost 30,000 Belgians excluded themselves from gambling venues in 2017 (Casino News Daily, 2018). Even the UK Parliament's Culture, Media and Sport Committee (2012) report on the workings of the 2005 Gambling Act, generally a model of complacency, recommended a universal self-exclusion system which would enable customers to self-exclude from all forms of gambling regulated by the Gambling Commission. GamStop, which aimed to do that for online gambling, started up a few years later, and by January 2019, 50,000 people were already reported to have registered with the scheme (iGaming Business, 2019a). The Commission's figures for 2015 to 2018 show the experience among gamblers of ever having self-excluded to be running at a rate of about 6%. The figure is higher for younger adults and highest, at over 10%, in the 25-to-34 year-old age group (Gambling Commission, 2019b).

But the main reason for highlighting self-exclusion here is because of what it says about modern gambling. Self-exclusion is a strange feature of the world of gambling, illustrating well its potential for creating addiction. The point about it for the present discussion is not whether it works – many do believe it can be very helpful for individuals and their families – but rather its significance in illustrating so pointedly that gambling is no ordinary commodity. It is a dangerous form of consumption that can trap people to the point where they have to take special steps to reduce the harm it is causing. There is no equivalent to self-exclusion in the ordinary world of purchaser–provider relations. There is no suggestion that a clothes store like Marks & Spencer, as part of good customer relations, should make it known to me that I can self-exclude myself from purchasing socks in the future if I feel I need to. M&S has no such policy as far as I know. The idea is ludicrous. Providing gambling and making a profit out of it is no ordinary business activity and should not be treated as such.

Interestingly enough, there is no direct equivalent to self-exclusion in the case of other recognised addictions either. What there most certainly is, however, is a whole host of ways in which people who are addicted to substances such as alcohol, heroin or crack cocaine try to fight their addictions, including using various tactics to distance themselves from temptation. It seems that partly for historical reasons, and perhaps in part because it is logistically easier to manage in the case of gambling, self-exclusion has achieved the status of being one of the best known and most widely supported addiction-control tactics for gambling. One of its special features is that it represents a collaboration between a person wishing to control temptation and the provider of the tempting product. This is surely an admission on the part of the provider and regulator that the product is indeed a dangerous one.

Gambling addiction now recognised

But, it may reasonably be asked, how can people lose control over their gambling to the point at which they need to resort to this strange tactic of requesting that the provider of the commodity they have been buying ban them from making further purchases? How can I justify my argument that ordinary people, including you and I, could find ourselves in that position – that we are all at risk because of the nature of the product itself and the way it is sold to us? I believe the best way of understanding this is to listen carefully to the accounts of their experiences given by people who know about it at first hand.

Addiction is not the only way in which gambling exacts a cost for society and its citizens, as we shall see in the next chapter. But, in my view, understanding that gambling is addictive is central to the debate about how society should deal with gambling. Rather than being any ordinary commodity like clothing, it is instead a dangerous one because it has the potential to create an addictive attachment which is harmful and difficult to break. This is not to say that all gambling is an addiction. In the same way as many people who drink alcoholic beverages are not addicted to alcohol consumption, so too is it the case that many people who engage in gambling are not addicted to it. Nor are all forms of gambling equally addictive: buying tickets for a national lottery is not as dangerous as playing roulette in a casino, engaging with a powerful modern electronic gambling machine (EGM) or placing complex sporting bets online. What is true, however, is that all types of gambling carry to some degree the potential for addiction.

One of the earliest personal testimonies, written in 1525 by Jerome Cardano, a Renaissance physician, astrologer, mathematician and writer, was well ahead of its time in recognising that gambling could become what he called 'a settled habit' amounting to an illness (Brenner & Brenner, 1990, p 139):

> During many years I have played not on and off but, I am ashamed to say, every day. Thereby I have lost my self-esteem, my worldly goods and my time. . . . Even if gambling is altogether evil, still, on account of the very many large numbers that play, it would seem to be a natural evil. For that reason, it ought to be discussed by medical doctors like one of those incurable diseases.

It was several hundred years before the experts understood this. An important event was the inclusion in 1980 of 'pathological gambling' in the American Psychiatric

Association's (APA) Diagnostic and Statistical Manual (DSM) of mental disorders, which is generally considered one of the most authoritative compendiums of mental health problems and their symptoms. Since then there has been some confusion about whether the DSM should include pathological gambling as an impulse-control disorder or as an addiction. The fifth revision of DSM, published in 2014, at last included 'gambling disorder', in the category Addiction and Related Disorders. The World Health Organisation (WHO) also now recognises gambling disorders, which are included, along with substance use disorders, in the 11th edition of its International Classification of Diseases (APA, 2014; WHO, 2018).

In fact, it has long been my view that gambling addiction, far from being one that might slowly and reluctantly be admitted to the accepted set of addictions, is actually the very clearest example of addiction. As the varieties of substances that it was recognised could lead to addiction grew in number from the 1970s onwards, it became clear that our understanding of addiction had to cope with substances with very different pharmacologies (Chandler & Andrews, 2018). Older theories of addiction, based on the effects on the brain of chronic ingestion of certain substances, started to give way to newer theories based on the effects of repetitive engagement in strongly rewarding, state-of-emotional-consciousness-changing activities, of which consumption of certain substances are examples, but so too is gambling. It seemed to me that we had been led astray in focussing on alcohol, nicotine, heroin, later cocaine and crack, then methamphetamine, cannabis, and later prescribed opiates and a plethora of new substances, legal and illegal. I am not alone in viewing gambling addiction as the prototype addiction. A group of cognitive scientists from South Africa and the USA had this to say (Ross *et al.*, 2008, pp 13, 16, 163–4):

> gambling is an ideal candidate to serve as the basic model of addiction in general . . . it provides the cleanest window on addiction. . . . This has been obscured by the cultural accident . . . that scientific study of addiction began by focusing on drugs . . . we see the intrinsic chemical properties of drugs as special-case *distractions* from the fundamental structure of addiction.

Later in this chapter I will try to summarise where the experts have got to in understanding the fundamental nature of addiction of which gambling addiction is a prime example. First, however, I want to devote a substantial section of the chapter to hearing at first hand from those who have experienced gambling addiction and can tell us what that is like. First-person accounts of gambling and other addictions have tended to be downplayed in the scientific literature (O'Connor, 2019) in favour of behavioural and neuroscientific forms of understanding. But the latter can be criticised for being mechanistic and reductionist (Murphy & Smart, 2019; Tekin, 2019). They can leave one dissatisfied, particularly perhaps because they give little room for one of the main things that comes across from first-person accounts, namely the intensely emotional nature of the experience of being addicted.

Real stories of gambling addiction

Many people who have developed a problem with their gambling, and then recovered from it, have written about it in one form or another, whether at book length, in articles, on websites or in some other way. I'll begin by drawing on three book-length accounts, all by men (more from women later). Each provides detailed, almost textbook examples of some of the main aspects of gambling addiction. They are Justyn Larcombe's, *Tails I Lose: the Compulsive Gambler Who Lost his Shirt for Good* (2014), Tony Kelly's *Red Card: The Soccer Star Who Lost It All to Gambling* (2013), and *Win, Lose, Repeat: My Life as a Gambler* (2017) by Chris Stringman. Justyn was fortunate in one respect. Most men with gambling problems, like Tony and Chris, started gambling early in life, as teenagers, but Justyn was a comparatively late starter, in his 40s, whose sports gambling escalated to a troubling level quite quickly – a pattern, often referred to as 'telescoping', thought to be more characteristic of women's gambling problems (and women's drug addiction, too), although this gender difference may be becoming less evident (Prever & Locati, 2017). One thing all three have in common is that, besides their gambling, each was a competent, successful member of society. Justyn Larcombe had been a Major in the army and later the youngest managing director in a large insurance business. Tony Kelly was a successful footballer, and Chris Stringman was a schoolteacher with a degree in economics.

Other sources I shall draw on include the book *Women and Problem Gambling* by Liz Karter (2013), a therapist who has specialised in working with women with gambling problems who provides a number of detailed examples of women addicted to playing gambling machines in arcades, buying scratchcards, or gambling online, for example; research that has involved in-depth interviews with people with gambling addiction in Scotland (33 men and 17 women were interviewed up to four times over a five-year period: Reith & Dobbie, 2012), England (a report of one of their studies from the International Gaming Research Unit at Nottingham Trent University – one of the few places to have a lengthy tradition of including studies that involve interviewing gamblers in some depth: Wood & Griffiths, 2007) and Australia (Carroll *et al.*, 2013; Hing *et al.*, 2016); and analyses of postings on websites that cater for people with such problems – one consists of over 100 comments, varying in length from one liners to one-page stories, taken from Finnish online gambling discussion forums, another of the first 500 postings on my own Gambling Watch UK (GWUK) website (Orford, 2018).

Although even these first-person accounts are still just snapshots of what is a complex and often long, drawn-out process, I believe they provide between them some understanding of what it is like to be addicted to gambling. In what follows, I have chosen to highlight just five elements of the experience, each of them elements which recur time and again. A further most important element which is notably missing here is any account of how people recovered from their gambling addictions. It has been shown in many studies now that people can and do recover from gambling addiction, as they do from other addictions, but that is beyond the scope of this chapter and this book. My purpose here is to illustrate what gambling addiction feels like when one is in the heat of it.

Preoccupation

The first thing that jumps out at one is the experience of gambling having become an overwhelming preoccupation that absorbs time and energy. Chris Stringman's (2017, pp 220–21) account contains a vivid picture. He writes about placing bets

> sitting on the toilet, stuck in traffic, squeezed into a standing room only train or bus . . . before and after work and, eventually, during work too. Worktime and free time then becomes a blur as any conceivable time just becomes gambling time . . . whilst eating . . . even . . . whilst having a shower. . . . I am ashamed to admit that I have placed bets whilst teaching. Set the kids some task, they return to their desks and you return to yours – with that computer on it.

There are numerous examples in Liz Karter's (2013, p 45) book of women experiencing the same intensity to their gambling. Here are two:

> At least then, I could go home. I had to stop. I was exhausted, I hadn't eaten or been to the toilet in hours. I'd had enough, but I knew if I won any more, I'd have kept gambling. I can never walk away with money.
>
> I stayed there all day. All day. When I got home, I had blisters on my fingers from pressing the buttons. I hate it, but I kept winning, telling myself I'd leave in five minutes and who am I kidding?

From the Gambling Watch UK website, a man in his late 20s:

> I find myself up every night dreaming of winning big or being able to predict what horse or football team will win. Scrolling through Facebook looking at all the big wins from football today on the tipster pages and just getting angry that you can't do that. It has completely taken over my life. All I think about is gambling or why didn't I back that or I was going to do that. Always finding an excuse.

The distorting effect that it has on one's thinking

Another hallmark of gambling addiction (as for other addictions), which people can describe once in the calmer waters of recovery from it, is the distorting effect that it has on one's thinking. People like Justyn, as rational as anyone else in the past and still so in other aspects of life, writes about having started to think in weird and harmful ways. He describes how he started to make decisions which could be explained to his wife and to himself as sensible but which with hindsight he can see were largely dictated by the need to make it easier to gamble. For example, he asked his employer if he could work more from home, which enabled him to spend more time gambling on his computer. He sold the house and rented, ostensibly to put him and his wife in a good position to look for a new house to buy, but the money that would have been used as a deposit for a new home was soon spent on gambling. To top it all, he managed to transfer money that his wife had inherited from her family into his account, not touching it for gambling to begin with but giving in to the temptation little by little as time went on.

There are also several places where he describes his state of mind and his confusion, recognising at one level that what he was doing was wrong and endangering so many things he valued. For example, he describes borrowing money off a long-standing good friend and off his mother, in both cases lying about what he needed the money for; selling things such as a valuable set of cartoons, his special army leaving gift – his Sword of Honour – and an ornament that had been a gift from his wife's father, all sold cheaply for instant money. All the while, he was convincing himself that he was still in control and could pay off his debts.

Tony Kelly (2013, pp 99–100) too believes he was not thinking straight:

> There should have been alarm bells ringing, as the more I gambled the bigger the effect on my behaviour and the worse my mood swings. . . . Somehow I still did not feel I was an addict, even though I was gambling regularly and paying the price in more ways than one.

He then recounts making foolish career decisions: for example, choosing to change clubs, ostensibly for good career reasons, but really in order to get the signing-on fee to finance his gambling. Making the bad decision to leave well-placed club Stoke City, he then began 'a bumpy but unstoppable slide down the football ladder'.

Liz Karter's clients were also aware that, as their gambling habit deepened, their thinking went awry. Her book is full of examples of her women clients having stolen or 'borrowed' money to finance their gambling, their gambling having left them too confused and lacking in energy and motivation to do anything else.

Justyn and Tony each describe in graphic detail examples of the kind of 'chasing of losses' that has so often been spoken about as a hallmark of gambling addiction, both making increasingly rash bets in the hope of big wins enough to settle the six-figure debts they had accumulated (not all addicted gamblers have large debts, but many I have heard from do, and they can be colossal).

One feature, often remarked on by gamblers in recovery, is a view of money that (Stringman, 2017, p 211):

> becomes almost bizarre. The gambler will try to spend as little as possible outside of gambling. . . . Only when you come out of gambling do you start to properly reassess the value of money but to reconnect with its true value is one of the hardest things for a reformed gambler to get their head round.

Secrecy

Secrecy and deceit are features of all addictions but no more so than in the case of gambling addiction. Tony Kelly, after counselling and his partner's and parents' support that he writes very positively about, admits, 'they never really knew the full extent of my problem'. Chris Stringman (pp 230, 232) too:

> Betting is a secretive activity. . . . You can sneak into the betting shop and no one from the outside can see you in there. . . . You can't reveal it to anyone, not least your partner . . . the deceit kills you, not being able to share it kills you. But you remain on your own.

From an Australian interview study (Hing *et al.*, 2016, p 41):

> I don't tell them [the family] anything and I have a million and one excuses of where the money went or why I've got, how I got this, and why this is not paid. So it's basically being devious because I don't want them to look at me and think – I don't even want their pity. . . . I just want them to think of me, same as others would be.

The desire to keep one's gambling secret from others is especially prominent in women's accounts. From the same study (p 42), one woman had not told her husband about the problem, 'Because I don't like to admit that I have a problem and . . . I like to think that, you know, I can control it'; and another had not disclosed her relapse:

> It's a struggle because you just don't feel confident enough to be raising the issues, you relapse, and all that . . . and you go, "Oh, I really don't wanna be a joke or I don't wanna look like I'm an idiot so I'm just gonna shut my mouth and hope it goes away".

One woman who took part in the Scottish study (Reith & Dobbie, 2012, p 515) described the lengths she went to to hide the extent of the gambling debts:

> I used to walk up the street and meet the postman in the morning, get the mail off him before it came through the letterbox. The sight of the postman was pure terror to me in case he [her husband] got a letter. He didn't know about anything. I had a pile of letters like that in unpaid bills and everything.

Personality change, guilt and shame

It is the effect of addiction on personal relationships which is often the most devastating. Justyn Larcombe (p 156) talks in his moving book about something which people who have experienced addiction are often horrified to have to admit: their

personalities had changed and they seemed to have become selfish and uncon-
cerned about others:

> Over the last year I had learned to hide my emotions, win or lose; to bury my
> feelings, to block out my conscience and blunt my instincts. I was also taking
> decisions based on my gambling habits and not for any other logical reason.
> I had turned into a selfish, self-centred cruel person who lacked a sense of
> humour and any feeling for anyone other than myself. . . . I realized I had
> become a different person, unrecognizable from the one I had been twelve
> months ago. I didn't like the new me.

From a posting on the Gambling Watch UK website:

> When I think back on my life, I could cry . . . what a waste! . . . chasing rain-
> bows all my days, looking for that big win! . . . not realising I had the big win
> all the time . . . my life, my family, my friends . . . no! The lure of gambling
> came first . . . what an arsehole I was. . . . I cringe thinking back to all the
> 'strokes' I pulled to get money to gamble . . . the lies, the deceit, stealing . . .
> my poor parents . . . then my wife . . . and yes my kids as well . . . gambling
> had a vice like grip on me . . . money lenders, pawn shops, ducking & diving,
> living on your wits, and being totally oblivious to the carnage and damage
> you left in your wake.

Karter's book too is full of examples of her women clients becoming 'preoccupied,
withdrawn and secretive'. One woman (p 60) was said to have returned from playing casino slot machines

> physically shaking, nauseous, unable to force down food or to sleep; wracked
> with shame, and guilt at time spent away from her children, and her marriage,
> yet again on the point of physical collapse, caused by all money being lost.

Another (p 122), at her lowest point, with hardly enough money to eat for the week,
let alone to pay bills or a babysitter, told Karter how she had crept out of the house
at night to go to the arcade, leaving her children

> sick with terror that they might wake up and discover her gone, or that
> someone else might discover she had left them alone, and yet her craving for
> gambling was so great that it felt as if she had no choice.

Like several others she regularly had suicidal thoughts.

Anna, addicted to the pokie machines in Victoria, Australia, attending a story-
writing workshop for problem gamblers and those at risk of problem gambling,
wrote about the intense feelings of shame that people with gambling problems
often describe (Bardsley, 2013, p 14):

The companion we gamblers all share is Shame and it keeps us there, keeps us quiet, we cannot speak out because Shame keeps us dumb. Keeps us in the zone, brings us back again and again, it is a crucial part of the cycle.

One Australian study found that problem gamblers seeking treatment commonly referred to their feelings of shame along with other terms such as 'embarrassed', 'weak', 'stupid', 'guilty', 'disappointed' and 'remorseful' (Carroll *et al.*, 2013), also believing that the public saw problem gamblers as 'stupid', 'foolish', 'weak', untrustworthy', 'secretive', 'losers', 'self-indulgent', 'lacking self-control', 'irresponsible', 'pathetic', 'desperate', 'lacking intelligence' and 'no hopers'. For example, one man feared other people would define him solely as a 'problem gambler':

> It makes you think that they're looking at you and seeing that weakness and perhaps that's all they're ever going to see after that and they're never going to be able to see you as successful or well-rounded and everything else.

The divided self

Once gambling has taken hold, it becomes a highly emotionally charged activity. The following quotation from Justyn Larcombe (p 132–33) nicely illustrates the conflict he found himself in and the conflicting emotions he felt.

> When I lost . . . I experienced feelings that were new to me. I felt self-loathing. How could I have been so stupid? I also felt anger that someone had taken *my* money, money I could have spent on my family, on a holiday or a present. . . . And I felt depressed. My life that had once been so good, so successful and fulfilled, was now reduced to this: secretly betting at home on a Monday morning, watching TV when everyone else was working hard to earn an honest wage. I hated those feelings. I could hardly bear another second of such self-loathing. I looked about desperately for anything that would restore my equilibrium and somehow give me back my self-respect and a sense of normality. The commentator was announcing the next game. As soon as I placed that second big bet, the dark feelings left me and were instantly replaced with hope. I felt alive again, the adrenaline was pumping through me, my parachute was on, and we were nearing the drop zone. This time I was sure to win. Ever the optimist, I settled back to watch. What a great way to spend a Monday morning! Everyone else was at work, slaving away. I could make money and enjoy myself at home.

As he so well describes it, the experience is a cyclical one of thinking about gambling, trying to resist it, getting excited about it in his case (a feeling of relief or numbness for others), and getting depressed afterwards. Like Justyn, Tony too describes, 'a roller-coaster ride through all the emotions from exaltation to total despair'. Much the same kind of emotional cycle is described by people who have a binge eating disorder or a substance addiction.

Many of us who have talked at length to people with gambling problems have been struck by the way in which people who have got into trouble with their gambling often draw a distinction between their problematic gambling and their 'real' selves, seeing gambling almost as an external force controlling them. For example, interviewed as part of the Scottish study (Reith & Dobbie, 2012, p 514), a male machine gambler said,

> I can feel the gambling coming on, you know. . . . You get taken over with the addiction and, eh, I'm just in a different world. . . . You're just oblivious to everything that is happening around you. . . . How can I explain that feeling? It's eh, you know you've got to do something, you don't want to do it. . . . I know I don't want to gamble but I've got to do it, cause I need to do it . . . it makes me do things I don't want to do.

The gambling self, the less 'real' or 'authentic' self, was described by participants in deeply negative terms, many talking of hatred, disgust, shame and self-loathing. For example another man (p 515) said,

> I see myself as this Golam-like creature crawling around through the night, snivelling, wanting money, thieving, grasping and yet I'm not like that at all – when I'm not gambling . . . I'd like to see myself as quite a nice reasonable bloke but then I have this other persona that I don't like very much.

Women in particular often described a profound sense of fear that their secret 'gambling self' might be revealed, feelings that frequently led to thoughts of suicide. There is a parallel here with the concept of the 'divided self' that has been used when talking about alcohol problems (Denzin, 1987).

Part and parcel of this agonising inner conflict is the way in which the motivation to gamble changes when people develop gambling problems, in the process deepening the sense that one is no longer gambling as one once was, nor any longer able to exert the control one once had. For example, Ben (not his real name), a horses, dogs and football gambler, who took part in the Nottingham Trent study (Wood & Griffiths, 2007, p 113), said,

> Gambling was an escape for me. It was an escape from the life that gambling had caused me. In the end gambling was the only escape I could escape from gambling [sic]. Does that make sense? . . . the only place I felt comfortable was in a betting shop

Justyn Larcombe too describes how his motivation to gamble had changed. Although he was still gambling to try and win back money, he recognised that 'gambling had become something more than that . . . a place where I could escape . . . my medication, anaesthetic for the horrible reality of the life I had created'. This kind of gambling to cope with negative emotions, emotional-coping gambling or gambling as 'self-medication', is often said to be more a common feature of women's gambling. In her book, Liz Karter concluded that gambling was providing women with an absorbing emotional escape from difficulties in their family or work lives, albeit a temporary escape and one that turned out to cause many more problems than it solved. As one woman said, 'It feels like hiding under the duvet – that kind of feeling that the world can't get at you'.

An even more common type of motivational change that people describe is an apparent loss of the original motivation for gambling. When addiction takes hold, it is common to hear people say that they lose interest in whatever it was about the substance or the activity that they previously found so pleasurable. One of the statements taken from the Finnish online gambling discussion forums: 'There is no meaningful experience of motivation, just the force of the habit itself'. The Nottingham Trent study found that many had realised they were now gambling for the sheer experience of gambling. As Tyrone, an off-course better in his early 20s, said (Wood & Griffiths, 2007, p 115),

> You are always looking or thinking that you're always going to get a big win to sort everything out and stuff like that. That is always in the back of my mind anyway. It didn't become about the money. It just became about gambling, just the whole thing of gambling.

Current scientific understanding of gambling and other addictions

From my reading of those and other first-person accounts and having listened to others, I believe those five characteristics – preoccupation, distorted thinking, secrecy, personality change and feelings of divided self – are central to the experience of gambling addiction. That list of five features is not quite the same as the rather dry, techno-medical list of symptoms to be found in the APA or WHO diagnostic handbooks, important though they are. But between them, understanding about those five agonising features does a better job of helping me understand what a grim, emotionally charged experience gambling addiction must be.

In the remainder of the chapter, I try to summarise where I think addiction science has got to in trying to fathom what gambling addiction is. Since gambling addiction is a good, even perhaps a prototypical, example of addiction, this is in large part the question of what addiction is.

Gambling addiction as a conditioned habit

My own starting point when trying to explain addiction is that it is in essence a habit, albeit a strong and seriously harmful one (Orford, 1985, 2001). But I am aware that such an apparently simple conceptualisation of addiction doesn't satisfy everyone. A disadvantage of that way of thinking of it lies in the fact that most people, including some experts, do not appreciate how strong habits can be, dismissing mere 'habit' as insufficient to the task of describing something as debilitating as addiction. An advantage, on the other hand, is that habit may go some way to understanding a central paradox of addiction, that it refers to actions that seem to be at the same time both voluntarily chosen and very difficult to resist. Habit does a good job of reconciling free choice and determination. William James (1891), often described as the father of psychology, famously wrote of the importance of forming and re-forming good habits as a necessary precondition for freedom. He thought of habits as half-conscious patterned acts that are neither completely automatic nor completely willed. Likewise, fellow pragmatist John Dewey (Valverde, 1998) thought that habits were 'precisely those patterns of action that are neither fully willed nor utterly determined, occupying that space in between perfect autonomy and utter necessity'. As the personal accounts given earlier illustrated, it is that paradox, that continued consumption appears to be undertaken voluntarily but at the same time feels out of one's control – the very hallmark of addiction in fact – which addicted gamblers experience as so confusing and demoralising.

Marc Lewis (2015), a neuroscientist who was himself 'a drug addict through most of my twenties', is one who shares my understanding of addiction as a habit, one that has become 'entrenched . . . a nasty, often relentless habit. A serious habit . . . a frightful, devastating, and insidious process of change in our habits'. The brain, he says, 'is a habit-forming machine'.

Another advantage of seeing gambling addiction as a habit disorder is that it fits well with what we know about the way in which gambling behaviour is rewarded, or 'reinforced', with wins, near misses and losses disguised as wins, encouraging the 'illusion of control', and in the various other ways discussed in Chapter 5. In order to comprehend how it is that gambling can take such a hold of a person's motivation it is necessary to appreciate how powerful conditioning can be, starting with the kind of 'reward conditioning' first studied by behavioural psychologists like B F Skinner several decades ago. Because money can be exchanged for so many things of value, and is therefore such a powerful 'generalised rein-forcer' of behaviour, gambling for money and winning has great capacity for shaping future behaviour. There are several features of gambling, particularly of certain forms of gambling, that increase its conditioning potential. One is the immediacy of receiving winnings: immediate consequences are much more effective in shaping behaviour than are delayed consequences. A more recent way of explaining the same thing uses the language of the newer science of behavioural economics. According to that way of thinking, the allure of immediate rewards can be explained in terms of 'delay discounting' whereby the subjective value of monetary or other reward diminishes with delay, in fact falling off very quickly with quite small delays (Bickel et al., 2007).

Another factor is the 'schedule of reinforcement'. B F Skinner commented back in the 1950s that the proprietors of gambling establishments were well aware of the power of what he called 'variable reward (VR) schedules' to instil patterns of behaviour that were very difficult to break. In fact, looked at from the perspective of that type of behavioural psychology, gambling operates on a variant of the powerful VR schedule, termed a random reinforcement or RR schedule, which is particularly habit-forming (Knapp, 1997). The 'volatility' of outcomes in modern gambling, also discussed in Chapter 5, is a different way of expressing the same thing. The uncertainty of a win, the high likelihood of winning something if one continues, however much one might lose in the process, not to mention the speed with which bets can be placed or machines spun, renders modern forms of gambling as addiction-creating devices.

Any account of gambling habit development must also include a role for stimulus conditioning, otherwise known as 'incentive conditioning' or 'classical conditioning', first studied by Ivan Pavlov. The act of gambling is always surrounded by stimuli of various kinds which, as habit develops, become conditioned by association, taking on some of the same rewarding properties and thereby acting as incentives in themselves – although the notion that responses to conditioned stimuli (CS) are somehow automatic has now given way to the idea that CS signal the availability or expectancy of reward which provokes physiological changes, craving and compulsion to engage with the object of one's addiction (Hogarth, 2019). Gambling settings are full of stimulating light and colour effects, sounds and other devices for drawing attention to winning, spinning reels and race commentaries. As one young British man with an addiction to gambling machines said, 'Although winning money was the first thing that attracted me to playing fruit machines, this was gradually converted to lights, sounds and excitement' (Griffiths, 1993). One of the best descriptions of this is contained in Dostoevsky's (1866) autobiographical novel *The Gambler* in which the main character Aleksey Ivanovitch describes how, when approaching the gambling hall, 'as soon as I begin to hear the clinking of money being poured out, I almost go into convulsions'. Dostoevsky – often described as the most famous compulsive gambler of all time – must himself have been very familiar with these feelings. Because these otherwise neutral cues become reinforcing in themselves, they play a vital role in maintaining behaviour such as betting despite the fact that much of the time the act of placing a bet results in financial loss rather than gain. Professional footballer Tony Kelly (2013, p 62) says,

> Looking back now it sounds ridiculous, but I can hardly begin to describe the buzz I got from walking into a bookie's. Every time I saw those Mecca Bookmakers red and green stripes I felt I wanted to take up their invitation to go inside.

The neuroscience of addiction

Work on neuroscience and gambling is a young but growing area of research which gives us another angle on why gambling might be so rewarding and habit-forming. A number of studies have now shown that the effects of gambling on the brain are similar in important respects to those of drugs such as amphetamine, cocaine, nicotine and alcohol. For example, it has been shown that uncertainty about the receipt of a reward, winning money on a gambling game and experiencing a near miss during a simulated machine gambling game, all produce effects in the limbic midbrain area – an area of the brain which is 'old' in evolutionary terms – which has been shown to be important for understanding drug habits and which is known to be involved in the control of motivation and emotion (Clark *et al.*, 2009). One specific area known as the striatum, especially part of it known as the accumbens, is particularly important. At one time this area was thought to be the brain's 'reward centre' which would become activated whenever reward was received. That idea has come to be replaced by a view of its function as a 'motivational core' which 'control[s] attention, perception, feeling and action', 'connecting actions with goals' (Lewis, 2015). However that is understood, there is general agreement amongst neuroscientists working on addiction that, in terms of neurochemistry, the release of the neurotransmitter dopamine is of central importance (Chandler & Andrews, 2018). But it is becoming ever more obvious that the brain is a very complicated organ with multiple connections between different regions and multiple pathways along which dopamine acts. Other areas such as the amygdala and insular areas may also play important roles in addiction.

One notion, first introduced by neuroscientists Robinson and Berridge (2000) and now widely ascribed to, is that, as an addictive habit develops, what has happened is a strengthening of the 'incentive salience' of the addictive substance or activity, or an increased 'wanting' for it, which is not the same as 'liking', in extreme form compulsion rather than pleasure. This distinction is probably of the utmost importance for understanding the experience of addiction. Habits become entrenched not because the object of desire, craving, need or compulsion continues to be so much enjoyed or liked but because repeated experience of reward has shaped how the motivational system operates, focussing attention and action towards the 'wanted' objective. In the process the affected person becomes a 'biased information processor', attending disproportionately to cues associated with the object of desire; thinking about and planning action about the object becomes a preoccupation, crowding out other interests and activities.

A technical expression for trying to capture the essence of what addiction is might be 'incentive motivational state'. That term embraces the important aspect that a person's motivation has been skewed towards, or captured by, a particular object or class of objects which have acquired abnormally heightened incentive value for that person. Neuroscientists now emphasise the brain's 'plasticity', including the ways in which its motivational core learns from experience, entrenching habits, adaptive or maladaptive, good or bad. This is why gamblers like Justyn, Tony, Anna and others found that their relationship with gambling changed, leaving them mystified about where their heightened desire or 'wanting' for gambling was coming from. As one neuroscientist had it, these powerful incentives, strengthened by repetition and the brain's plasticity, are 'unsensed incentives' (Wise, 2002).

Midbrain dopamine projections to other brain areas include not only those within the complex midbrain region itself, where it is thought reward-driven motivation is controlled, but also projections to other areas, importantly those connecting the midbrain to the prefrontal cortex (PFC), particularly the latter's medial and dorsolateral areas (Lewis, 2015). One idea that has become widely accepted is that addiction can be explained as a transition from voluntary action to more automatic, habitual behaviour, represented in the brain as a transition from prefrontal cortical to midbrain striatal control of behaviour. It is as if our normally well-functioning planning system – the 'executive' if you will – has been overwhelmed by an 'impulsive', artificially created, powerful desire (Murphy & Smart, 2019). Neuroscientists sometimes talk of the brain's motivational system having been 'hijacked' by a powerful new attachment to a substance(s) or activity. As the South Africa–USA collaborative group colourfully put it, 'In effect, addiction first hijacks the reward system below decks, then commits mutiny on the bridge by sabotaging the cognitive systems that would otherwise check its influence' (Ross *et al.*, 2008).

Incidentally, much publicity has been given to the finding that the PFC matures gradually over a long period of time, only reaching full maturity in our mid-20s (Lewis, 2015). If addiction at the level of the brain can be thought of as a victory for the 'impulsive' over the 'reflective' in this competition between neural systems, this may go some way towards explaining why adolescents and young adults are most at risk of addictions of all sorts, including gambling.

The importance of conflict

Addictions, then, are habits, which can be very powerful, preoccupying and mystifying to the people experiencing them. What imparts to them their most terrifying aspect, however, is the fact that they come into conflict with a person's other interests, obligations, life plans and sense of right and wrong. If humans, with our capacity to learn from experience, are 'habit machines', then acquiring habits that serve us well and are consonant with the rest of a life that has coherence, is essential. But if along the way we are unlucky enough to fall prey to one of the potentially addictive habits, we can be in serious trouble. For me, one of the most perceptive ways of thinking of addiction, expounded by Levy (2006) in the *Canadian Journal of Philosophy*, sees it as a loss of full capacity to consistently plan and exert one's will across time. Agency is fragmented. Life loses its coherence. This takes us full circle, back to the popularity of self-exclusion for gamblers. Self-exclusion demonstrates as clearly as could be that addicted gamblers 'invest resources in both gambling *and* in efforts not to gamble or to gamble less' (Ross *et al.*, 2008). Addiction is strong habit in conflict with what one otherwise would and should be doing and struggles to do. One of the most serious facets of this conflict, this lack of coherence, is the dissonance felt by addicted gamblers between how they are thinking and behaving and how they believe they should be thinking and acting – a kind of 'moral injury', to use a term that is coming to be used in other contexts that can give rise to such feelings of dissonance (Wood, 2016) – which, as we saw earlier, is a source of shame, self-stigma and often suicidal thoughts.

I have always maintained that conflict is the principal hallmark of all addictions (Orford, 1985, 2001). Conflict is not a side effect of addiction, it is the essence of it. This is because of the state of motivational conflict brought about by such a rooted habit. Powerful appetitive habits such as a gambling addiction create harms such as financial loss, declining mental health and relationship difficulties. The anticipated immediate rewards of engaging in the addictive activity are then pitted against equally strong motives to use time and money for more essential purposes; to behave responsibly in the eyes of family, friends and work colleagues; and to behave in a way consistent with one's own standards and self-image.

Another way of conceiving of this is to think of one having a conflict of interests, in a sense at war with oneself, with now diminished capacity to consistently make choices regarding consumption which are in keeping with other life plans (Ainslie, 2011). Faced with opposing motives of such strength, the addicted person becomes an even more biased information processor, a 'harassed decision-maker', trying to hide one's behaviour from others, finding devious and perhaps illegal ways of obtaining money, becoming more defensive about behaviour, increasingly tense, guilty, beset with feelings of shame like Anna, confused, desperate and even suicidal. Resolutions to curb the behaviour are made and broken, and the behaviour becomes more compulsive. At the same time, the addicted gambler is increasingly likely to experience distress in the form of irritability, agitation, restlessness and depression, as well as psychosomatic symptoms such as headaches, insomnia, racing heart and shaking, associated with experiences of loss, feelings of indecision about continuing gambling and worry and preoccupation about debts and other costs of gambling.

I have termed this 'acute gambling distress'. I have heard gamblers describe it as 'gambling fever'. The repeated struggle over whether or not to gamble again is a central component and is itself emotionally draining. In fact a whole area of experimental psychology has developed around the idea of 'ego fatigue' (Baumeister, 1998): exerting effort to control temptation depletes one's capacity to concentrate on and perform well on other tasks. This is something that Gamblers Anonymous and other 12-step mutual help organisations have long understood: if you have a serious gambling compulsion, battling alone with the conflict whether to gamble or not is exhausting and unlikely to be consistently effective.

Ideas of conflict over behaviour are long-standing. An example is Aristotle's concept of *akrasia* (Pickard & Ahmed, 2019), the phenomenon of acting contrary to one's considered judgement about what course of action would be best. William James (1891) too was impressed, when it came to 'moral habits', by the idea of a conflict between 'two hostile powers'. The idea of the hijacked midbrain dopamine system in conflict with prefrontal cortical self-regulation, discussed above, can be seen as a theory of conflict at a neurological level. In fact, as prominent British addiction psychologist Nick Heather (2018) has pointed out, several modern lines of theory about addiction have close parallels with the philosophical idea of *akrasia*: delay discounting that uses the analogy of a personal struggle and a kind of intrapersonal 'bargaining' between succumbing to immediate temptation versus being ruled by longer term planning; dual-process decision theory which speaks of the conflict between the automatic, unconscious system 1 and the controlling, conscious, planning system 2; and ego- or resource-depletion theory (mentioned earlier).

What unites all of those approaches is the idea of two cognitive or motivational systems, or two brain systems, or two alternative sets of actions in opposition to one another. They share the idea that people when addicted are in a state of disunity about their behaviour and that much of what we see as addicted gambling behaviour can be understood as features of people in heightened conflict, in two minds about their behaviour, at war with themselves if you like.

Conclusion

In this chapter I hope I have been able to show that gambling addiction is now well established as a recognised form of addiction, in fact as one of the clearest forms of addiction.

A substantial part of the chapter was given over to hearing at first hand from those who have experienced gambling addiction and know what that is like. They illustrated the intensely emotional nature of the experience of being addicted to gambling; specifically the preoccupation with gambling, the distorting effect that it has on one's thinking, the secrecy that surrounds it, the feelings of guilt and shame, and the sense of a divided self.

The chapter went on to summarise my understanding about the fundamental nature of addiction of which gambling addiction is a prime example. I explained addiction as a strong, entrenched and seriously harmful habit. Studies of the neuroscience of addiction support that model. What is a central feature of the experience of gambling addiction, as for other addictions, is the fact that it comes into conflict with a person's other interests, obligations, life plans and sense of right and wrong. Life loses its unity, its coherence. This took us full circle, back to the popularity of self-exclusion for gamblers, a topic with which the chapter began. The strange phenomenon of gambling self-exclusion demonstrates clearly not only what a dangerous commodity gambling is but also how the experience of being addicted to it tears one in two.

I have tried to demonstrate how it is that we can become trapped in a gambling habit to the point at which the attachment is so strong that it overwhelms our usual capacity to reflect on our lives and to plan ahead as best we can. In the process we become no longer sure which is our real self. We now find it difficult to fathom our own behaviour. Our motivation for continuing to gamble has become more complicated to the point at which it is no longer obvious whether there is any motivation for it at all.

No wonder Justyn, Anna, Tony, Chris and so many others who have experienced gambling addiction at first hand found it such a devastating experience and wanted, afterwards, to tell others about it.

7

GAMBLING'S HARM TO INDIVIDUALS, FAMILIES, COMMUNITIES, AND SOCIETY

Addiction to gambling is a devastating condition and one that is more prevalent than most people realise. In Britain, the Gambling Commission estimated that in 2016 there were approximately 350,000 adults (16 years and over) with gambling problems (0.7% of all adults; more among men and 25-to-34 year-olds) and a further 550,000 whose gambling was putting them at 'moderate risk' (1.1%, again more men and 25-to-34s) (Gambling Commission, 2019b). There are no equivalent data for under-16s, but it is generally accepted that they are particularly at risk of experiencing problems with gambling if they are not protected from exposure to it (National Research Council, 1999; Orford et al., 2003). The fact that gambling, particularly in some of its modern commercialised forms, is responsible for addiction, is the strongest single argument against its thoughtless expansion. But the harm associated with gambling is not limited to addiction per se. In fact, focussing solely on addiction may play into Establishment hands. After all, part of the industry discourse is that their products are essentially safe. The only exception is that 'small minority' who suffer addiction, and they can be identified, re-educated or excluded – preferably self-excluded.

In this chapter I consider an alternative, public health approach to identifying the range of harms associated with gambling. This approach recognises the central importance of addiction and its effects on individuals but looks more widely at the harms occurring to the broader constituency of people as family members, citizens of towns and communities, and as concerned members of society more generally. In the context of gambling this is often referred to as the 'harms approach'. In some countries, such as New Zealand and Canada, it has been familiar for some years – although many believe that even in those countries it has been mostly honoured in name only. In my part of the world, Britain, it is comparatively new and is part of the growing backlash against the growth of gambling. It is an important step towards a more comprehensive public health approach to the subject.

One sign of this move was the appearance in 2018 of a significant report entitled *Measuring gambling-related harms: a framework for action* (Wardle *et al.*, 2018). It was the output of an expert group assembled to a) agree upon a definition of gambling-related harms to be used in British policy and practice, b) consider how gambling-related harms may be better understood, measured and monitored, and c) explore whether it is possible to attach some estimate of the social cost of gambling-related harms and make recommendations about how that may be done. It states clearly that gambling is a public health issue. The report breaks harms down into impacts on resources, relationships and health.

That report was very much influenced by the first serious attempt in another country, Australia, to list comprehensively the range of harms which gambling can give rise to, including what the World Health Organisation, in the context of an international project on alcohol-related harm, has called 'harms to others', or HtO (Casswell *et al.*, 2011). The Australian group (Langham *et al.*, 2016), based in Queensland, carried out a literature review and focus groups and interviews with a range of relevant professionals and with individuals who identified that they had experienced harm from either their own or someone else's gambling. Among the many types of gambling-related harm of which they found evidence, some were in the nature of acute crises, while others were those that were likely to continue to operate for long periods of time – what they called 'legacy' effects. They also recognised 'lifecourse and intergenerational harms' including loss of life course events such as marriage or having children, forced change of career, having to move home, homelessness and incarceration.

Table 7.1 provides a summary of the main areas of harm to be discussed briefly in this chapter.

The British group's third aim of trying to estimate the costs of gambling-related harms is more difficult. Another important report came out at the end of 2016. This was from the Institute for Public Policy Research (IPPR), an influential and progressive British thinktank. They calculated what they thought were the excess costs to Government associated with people having problems with gambling. These included the costs associated with mental health care, hospitalisation, providing jobseekers allowances, loss of tax income due to unemployment, and costs associated with homelessness and incarceration. Their best estimate of the total of those costs was somewhere between £260 million and £1.16 billion per year for Britain as a whole.

Because IPPR was cautious in making those estimates, the difference between its minimum and maximum estimates was obviously wide. Furthermore, IPPR was unable to take into account what most of us would consider the largest 'costs' of having a gambling problem – those that are more personal and less tangible, such as effects on one's state of mind, quite apart from any healthcare that is sought on account of it, and effects on family and other relationships. Nor were they able to take into account the harmful effects experienced by affected others such as partners, parents, children and other family members, co-workers and close friends. An attempt by economists to estimate the costs associated with problem

TABLE 7.1 A summary of some of the main areas of gambling's harm

Harm experienced by the person who gambles	Finances	Reduced disposable income/financial insecurity Debt and bankruptcy
	Work and education	Reduced work performance, absenteeism, job loss, reduced chances of finding work, effects on career progression
	Health and well-being	Addiction Mental ill-health Suicidal thoughts/suicide Decline in quality of relationships Poorer physical health
	Homelessness	Rough sleeping Housing insecurity
	Crime	Embezzlement, stealing goods at work or making fraudulent expense claims
Harm to affected family members and others	Financial	Family financial insecurity Loss of family savings Lifestyle/coping adjustments
	Relationships	Reduced reliance on/trust in the relationship Conflict/domestic abuse Separation Children may take on extra responsibilities including caring responsibilities
	Health and well-being	Anxiety, depression and other symptoms of stress Children at risk of effects on education and health
Harm to communities and society	Local communities	Changes to the character of an area Loss of local control over the amenities and nature of a community Impact on other local businesses Extraction of money from poorer areas Risks to an area's young and most vulnerable
	Society generally	Normalisation of gambling Contributes to inequality Contributes to a certain kind of society, perhaps helping undermine traditional values

gambling is not new (Grinols, 2003), but a strict economic view of 'costs' concentrates on the costs to the public purse and therefore excludes much of what might be thought of as the real costs of gambling for affected others, the community and wider society. The provision of treatment or court and police time would be treated as public costs, but family debt, for example, might be excluded from consideration on the grounds that it is simply a transfer of money from one person or group to another, a private rather than a public cost. But even so, the IPPR figures are frightening.

Harms experienced by those who gamble

Let us begin with those harms that refer explicitly to problems borne in the first instance by those who gamble excessively, harmfully. Those whose gambling is most likely to give rise to these harms are those who are addicted to gambling. Addiction and harm, although not precisely the same thing, are highly correlated. But, when adopting the wider public health 'harms' perspective, there are two points that need to be taken into account. One is something often referred to as the *prevention paradox*. Gambling addiction, or problem gambling to use the more general term, lies on a continuum. For every one person who, like those we heard from in Chapter 6, has developed a very serious addiction to gambling, there are several whose gambling is a problem, but to a lesser degree. However, because they are more numerous, paradoxically their gambling contributes a larger sum total of gambling-related harm. The other term to note is *attributable fraction*. For example, gambling is strongly related to debt, but not all debt can be attributed to gambling, even amongst those who are addicted to it. Epidemiologists are always cautious about this and rightly so.

Note also that, although these harms may be experienced most acutely by those who gamble, which is why they are discussed under this first heading, they are also likely to have harmful effects for family members and others and incur losses for the wider community in the form of costs to the public purse and in other ways. The categories of harm – to those who gamble, to families, colleagues, communities and society generally – are in reality not easily separable. All are harms and costs to us all.

Some of the most costly gambling-related harms experienced by those who gamble are the following. Much of the evidence is summarised in Sulkunen *et al.*'s (2019) international review.

Gambling-related debt and bankruptcy

Gambling can make a very significant contribution to individual debt and both temporary and persistent poverty (Barnard *et al.*, 2013). Personal debt has been recognised as a major and growing problem (Değirmencioğlu & Walker, 2015). Gambling, which nearly always results in losses, can only increase the problem. As has long been recognised, it can be due to borrowing money to spend on gambling; or due to taking out loans, often including expensive unsecured loans; or due to borrowing money to meet financial commitments which cannot otherwise be met due to gambling losses (Ladouceur *et al.*, 1994). Not all people with gambling problems are in debt, but many are, and often the size of the debts, which is correlated with the severity of the gambling problem, is stag-gering, as postings on my Gambling Watch UK website regularly attest. Studies conducted in the USA, Canada and Australia have found significant average current debts for those with gambling problems, with estimated averages rang-ing from US$2,500 to over US$50,000 depending on the sample (Sulkunen *et al.*, 2019).

Personal bankruptcy is more prevalent among people with gambling problems – an estimated lifetime prevalence of around 10% to 20% in some studies – although most of the evidence about this comes from the USA (Grinols, 2003). An associa-tion between gambling and personal bankruptcy is observed also at the community level; US counties and cities with major gambling facilities have significantly higher bankruptcy-filing rates than other areas. Most studies have also found that the opening of a casino or introduction of other forms of gambling in a community increases the rate of bankruptcies (Sulkunen *et al.*, 2019).

Homelessness

Nor is it surprising that having a gambling problem can affect one's ability to obtain housing or keep up rent or mortgage payments and can lead to homeless-ness and rough sleeping. A number of studies carried out with homeless people have found a high prevalence of problematic gambling, of the order of 10–15% in studies in the UK, USA and Australia, with an exceptionally high 39% recorded in one Australian study (Sulkunen *et al.*, 2019). The first British study on the subject (Sharman *et al.*, 2016) was carried out in the Westminster area of London. Over 400 people using services for homeless people were interviewed, and problem gambling prevalence was found to be 11%. The figure was higher still amongst rough sleepers compared to those living in hostel accommodation. This repre-sents a large group nationally who would have been completely missed by general population prevalence surveys and whose gambling problems are probably being missed by homelessness services much of the time.

Work-related problems, job loss and crime

Gambling-related problems can lead to reduced work performance, absenteeism, job loss and reduced chances of finding work (Lesieur, 1984). What Tony Kelly (2013) said about the effects of his gambling on his football career is a clear case in point (see Chapter 6). Online gambling during work time, which Chris Stringman (2017) described, has specifically been linked with loss of productivity, borrowing money from colleagues and requests for cash advances on salary. Gambling can lead to criminal acts, including embezzlement, stealing goods at work or making fraudulent expense claims. Impacts in the workplace may be particularly impor-tant at gambling venues since there is a relatively high prevalence of gambling problems among gambling sector employees (Sulkunen *et al.*, 2019).

Gambling-related crime in general is a broader issue for individuals and society, extending well beyond the workplace. It includes not only crimes committed by individuals in order to obtain resources for gambling or to cover gambling losses (Meyer & Stadler, 1999) but also the provision of illegal gambling, which is widespread in many parts of the world as discussed in Chapter 2, and fraud such as match-fixing in sports. The large amounts of money involved make it easier for organised and professional criminals to commit illegal acts such as money laundering, as well as other criminal activities such as prostitution, drug trading and illegal, online pornography which are frequently associated with gambling. Gambling venues can also attract street crime, police reports of incidents in the vicinity of British betting shops offering high-stake EGM gambling being an example. Gambling-related crime incurs obvious costs including police, court and prison costs (Banks, 2014; Sulkunen *et al.*, 2019).

Mental health problems and substance use

For some time, research, both in clinical and general population samples, has consistently been showing that people who experience problem gambling are more likely than others to also be experiencing mental health or substance problems (Petry, 2005). Among the most frequently reported mental health problems co-occurring with gambling problems, according to psychiatric research, are depression and anxiety disorders, including phobias and panic disorder. A variety of other co-occurring conditions have been reported, including attention deficit hyperactivity disorder, obsessive-compulsive disorders and schizophrenia. Such co-occurrence of problems, or 'comorbidity' to use the medical term, is associated with higher severity of illness and associated disability, increased rates of recurrence, delays in seeking help and slower recovery. But causality is complex. Problem gambling can cause or contribute to other disorders, or the other way round. It can also reflect other underlying disorders or common factors, or the two may be causally independent but reinforce and intensify one another with time (Sulkunen *et al.*, 2019).

Substance use disorders are the most common conditions co-occurring with problem gambling. Alcohol and tobacco dependence are, as is to be expected, the most commonly co-occurring substance problems, and both are linked to gambling at the level of individual problems and at the level of gambling events. People with gambling problems increase their smoking when gambling. They are also more likely than others to report being drunk or high while gambling. Gambling under the influence of alcohol results in larger bets and reduces the perception of consequences of risk-taking; and drinking while gambling has been linked to higher severity of gambling problems (Sulkunen *et al.*, 2019).

General health is also likely to be poorer among those experiencing gambling problems. Specifically, gambling has been found to be associated with taking less exercise, having more emergency hospital visits, and suffering more than others from a variety of physical health issues, including headaches, high blood pressure, cardiac arrest, arthritis, indigestion, weight loss, tachycardia, angina, cirrhosis and Parkinson's disease (Sulkunen *et al.*, 2019).

Suicide

Suicide is now recognised in the UK and elsewhere as a major cause of very premature death, particularly among young men. In the previous chapter, illustrations were given of the way in which having an addiction to gambling can make a person feel suicidal. Research since at least the 1990s has been confirming that people with gambling problems have elevated rates of suicidal thoughts, suicide attempts and actual suicides (Dickerson, 1990), and a growing body of evidence now links suicides directly to gambling. One of the comparatively early studies examined coroners' records in Victoria, Australia, for any mention of gambling (Blaszczynski & Farrell, 1998). Although such records were very incomplete on the subject then – as no doubt they still are – sufficient evidence was available in the cases they examined to conclude that there was strong support for a causal role for gambling. As they said at the time (p 94):

> Intuitively, it is reasonable to predict a strong causal relationship between excessive gambling and risk for suicide. . . . Under conditions of intense emotional distress, turmoil and sense of hopelessness, suicide is often considered as the only optional solution to their predicament.

It was already known in the 1990s that Las Vegas had the highest suicide rate in the USA both for residents and for visitors. High suicide rates had also been found in Atlantic City after casinos were opened there. The Las Vegas effect was confirmed in a report (Wray *et al.*, 2008) showing that the odds of suicide were 50% higher among Las Vegas residents than among residents elsewhere and that visitors to Las Vegas doubled their risk for suicide compared to those who stayed in their home county or visited another destination. Leaving Las Vegas was associated with a 20% reduction in risk for suicide. A Swedish study of over 2,000 people with health care diagnoses of gambling disorder in the years 2005 to 2016 found a mortality rate twice that expected and a rate of mortality by suicide 15 times that expected (Karlsson & Håkansson, 2018). On the basis of the limited evidence which exists, the active British campaign group Gambling with Lives, referred to in Chapter 1, has estimated that in the UK there could be in the region of 250 to 650 gambling-related suicides a year.

Family harm

Amongst the people who know most about the harm gambling can cause are close family members – the parents, partners, children, siblings and other relatives of those who are personally experiencing problem gambling. Yet in all the debate and discussion about gambling there has been an unfortunate tendency to neglect this group of 'affected others'. There are a lot of them. The 2010 British Gambling Prevalence Survey included the question: *In the last 12 months, has any close relative of yours (including partner) had a gambling problem?* In that representative British sample, 3.8% answered that question in the affirmative, which, multiplied out, produces an estimate of over one and a half million people in the country as a whole – and that was an adult survey, so it excludes children under 16 who have parents with gambling problems (Wardle *et al.*, 2011). From their surveys of large Australian samples, Goodwin *et al.* (2017) concluded that, on average, four to six others are affected whenever there is a gambling problem. Three main areas of family harm are financial harm, relationship harm and harm to family members' health and well-being (McComb *et al.*, 2009; Velleman *et al.*, 2015).

Financial harm

When the person with the gambling problem is an adult breadwinner, financial effects for the whole family often loom large. Amongst the financial harms for affected others listed by the authors of the Australian harms study (Langham *et al.*, 2016) are reduced capacity to purchase luxury items such as holidays, reduction of discretionary spending such as spending on children's sports, erosion of savings, the need to manage cash-flow problems by taking on additional employment, use of pawn and payday loan services, and inability to spend on such things as insurance, repairs or maintenance, which may result in delayed harms, or on items such as clothing, transport, accommodation or food, which will have more immediate consequences. The legacy consequences of such harms include continued financial hardship, reliance on welfare and restricted credit.

The often very serious financial harms of gambling for families have been documented in studies from many countries. They are well illustrated in the report of a study of 50 Singapore residents who were either seeking help for a relative with a gambling problem or had lodged an application for a casino-exclusion order (Mathews & Volberg, 2013). More than half of the families had substantial family debts, ranging from tens of thousands to hundreds of thousands of dollars. Family members often had to make lifestyle adjustments, for example spouses with childcare responsibilities being forced into employment or family members having to work night shifts or take extra jobs. A quarter reported having had to sell their housing. Harassment from loan sharks was often mentioned, including angry and abusive calls or unanticipated visits to the home demanding payment, plus threats of further consequences including harm to family members and children.

Because of the secrecy that often surrounds gambling, the extent of a family's financial difficulties may not be fully apparent to members of the family for some time. Once the scale of the financial problem is more fully out in the open, affected family members face a new set of 'coping dilemmas', as I call them (Orford, 2012). They may have to decide whether to cut back on their spending, which would impact on their lifestyle. They may make the difficult decision to take on the role of managing family finances and controlling the relative's access to money in order to either help the relative or to gain as much control as possible in order to protect the family's financial position. Taking on this role can be in itself highly stressful, adding to what is already a highly stressful set of circumstances. Family members may have to return to work, sell property and items that can no longer be afforded or make necessary changes in childcare or education (Velleman *et al.*, 2015).

Relationship harm

For many affected family members, it is the impact on relationships that is most deeply felt. The exact nature of the stress for family members naturally depends on the form of relationship, although most has probably been written about what it is like for partners, especially wives, of people who have gambling problems. Less has been written, for example, about what it is like for parents of adolescents or young adults with gambling problems, a situation I am personally familiar with.

One of the most detailed accounts of what it is like to be the spouse of some-one with a gambling problem is contained in the book *Betting Their Lives: The Close Relations of Problem Gamblers*, which reported the results of a study funded by the Ontario Problem Gambling Research Centre (Tepperman, 2009). One of the things that many spouses found most difficult were their gambling partners' mood swings.

> When he's leaving, he's very positive and upbeat. When he comes back, depending on how he fares, if he wins he's still up, if he loses he's down – he's angry, frustrated, you can't say two words to him and everything triggers anger.
>
> (p 179)

Loss of trust is a significant factor in relationships affected by problem gambling. Commonly, family members describe their gambling relatives as distant, uninterested and neglectful of family roles and responsibilities. They talk about having to 'tread carefully', not wanting to 'cause' further gambling behaviour. The Australian study (Langham *et al.*, 2016) listed reduced amount and quality of time spent with the person who gambles, dishonest communication, feelings of unequal contribution to the relationship, reduced engagement in family or social events with the person who gambles, conflict which can range from minor or occasional to major or constant, and disruption to other relationships due to the demands of trying to manage the relationship with the person who gambles. Legacy consequences include social isolation, ongoing resentment and feelings of guilt and shame, long-term damage or estrangement or distortion of relationship roles, and effects on future relationships, as well as ongoing engagement with a family court. It is no surprise that there is a much higher rate of divorce among couples affected by problem gambling than in the general population.

High rates of domestic abuse, both verbal and physical, have been reported in families where one member gambles excessively (Dowling *et al.*, 2016; Sulkunen *et al.*, 2019). As with other co-occurring problems, cause and effect is likely to be complex and will depend on a variety of factors, not least the sexes of and form of relationship between a person with a gambling problem and his or her affected family member. However, there can be little doubt that problem gambling, when it is present, increases family tension and the likelihood of domestic conflict.

Family members' health and well-being

There is a toll on family members' health and well-being. The initial disclosure or discovery of a gambling problem can itself be 'sudden, devastating and traumatic' (McComb *et al.*, 2009). Thereafter, family members describe a feeling of being on high alert, watching their relatives and trying to work out whether gambling is continuing, all of which leads them to feeling exhausted, more stressed and ineffectual. Family members often feel that they are alone in experiencing what they are going through. There is no guidance readily available about how best to cope. They may not know where to get the support they need. Particularly poignant is the guilt that many family members describe because they think they might be the reason for their relatives' gambling problems or because, despite their efforts, they have been unable to do anything to stop the behaviour: spouses often suffer self-doubt and guilt, 'carrying a mistaken sense of responsibility for the gambling relative's actions'. As one mother posted on the Gambling Watch UK website:

> My son is a gambler and I don't know how to help him. He goes to bookies, casinos, anywhere there are roulette machines. He has lost at least £15k of my money, besides his own. I'm at my wits end and desperately in need of help. I hate to see him so down and depressed. I feel I've failed him as a mom by not noticing earlier.

Among family member harms can be listed their feelings of frustration, anxiety, suspicion, distress, insecurity, shame, guilt and low self-worth, as well as the consequent increased risk of depression, anxiety and self-harm. There are also physical impacts for family members, such as tiredness, increased blood pressure, loss of sleep, migraine, reduced levels of self-care and consequent increased risk to physical well-being, higher incidence of disease or injury and exacerbation of other disorders. To add to the list are harms under the headings of reduced performance at work or study due to tiredness or distraction, absenteeism due to time spent managing problems of the person who gambles, and reduced availability for others outside the family. Others fall under the heading of criminal activity, not only as a result of being the victim of crime from the person who gambles but also due to increased vulnerability to engaging in crimes of opportunity or crimes of duress due to financial hardship and debt (Langham *et al.*, 2016; Velleman *et al.*, 2015).

The impact on children

Children are likely to be the most vulnerable of all family members affected by a gambling problem. One US expert (Lorenz, 1987) who looked into this in the 1980s observed:

> Children of the pathological gambler are probably the most victimized by the illness. . . . Emotionally and financially dependent upon the gambler during the worst of the illness, it is the children who are the most helpless. They hear the arguments, recriminations, apologies, broken promises, insults, lies, and fights. They hear their mother arguing with their father about not having money for food, clothes, or school items for the children.

Although there is still almost no recognition on the part of health and social services and policymakers about the experiences of children who live in families where an adult has a gambling problem, a number of relevant studies have been carried out in the USA and elsewhere. Two of them compared children with problem gambling parents with control groups of children. One found the children of problem gambling parents to be at much greater risk for health-threatening behaviours, such as smoking and alcohol or drug use, and for experiencing educational difficulties and emotional disorders, including depression and suicidal thoughts, and the other found they reported more depressive feelings and more conduct problems at mid-adolescence. They also experienced an increase in depressive symptoms from mid-adolescence to early adulthood. One asked about the young people's feelings concerning their parents' gambling. Two-thirds reported feeling sad and over half emotionally hurt, depressed and confused, with between a quarter and a half feeling angry most or all of the time, pity for their parents' gambling, hateful, shameful, helpless, isolated, abandoned and guilty (Jacobs *et al.*, 1989; Vitaro *et al.*, 2008).

Children may find themselves having to take on parent-like, caring or other responsibilities inappropriate for their age (Langham *et al.*, 2016). Family financial pressure means some have to start work early in life, having to work alongside their schooling, or having to support themselves during post-secondary education, sometimes needing to make career decisions that they might not otherwise have taken. Children in the Singapore family study constantly compared themselves with others who had come from good financial backgrounds, found it hard to adapt and experienced substantial distress as a result (Mathews & Volberg, 2013).

The various financial, relationship, health and well-being and other harms to which affected family members are liable have 'life course and intergenerational' consequences for themselves and their families, including children. These include delay in the occurrence of normal life course events, continuing financial insecurity, forced moves, and loss of relationships and social connections (Langham *et al.*, 2016).

Effects for others beyond the family

In summary, the experience of being a family member of a close relative who is gambling problematically can be described as one of powerlessness (Langham *et al.*, 2016; Orford, 2013). Addiction erodes autonomy, and the disempowerment it entails is contagious, rippling out to others, to close family members and beyond. Extended family members, close friends and colleagues can also be affected, and their relationships and joint projects harmed. The Australian Productivity Commission (1999), in its comprehensive assessment of the costs and benefits of gambling to Australian society, concluded, on the basis of a survey of clients in counselling, that on average a single gambling problem adversely affected no less than seven other people. To take just one of many possible examples, the managers and fellow team members of professional footballers with gambling problems (Lim *et al.*, 2016) are likely to experience some of the same harms known to close family members; for example, witnessing the threat to their effectiveness as a team and feelings of powerlessness and uncertainty about how to cope with what they are seeing.

Harms to town centres and communities

The main railway station in Birmingham, where I have lived and worked for over 20 years, has been undergoing major renovation. Its new main entrance was opened while I was planning the writing of this book. Directly opposite is a multi-fronted betting shop run by one of the big betting chains. Turn to the right and you will find within just a few yards another two betting shops run by its competitors. Quite apart from what this indicates to rail travellers about the image of Britain's second city, it nicely illustrates the problems that have been taxing local councillors and officials and Members of Parliament for some time, particularly those representing poorer areas. What has been concerning them are the apparent proliferation, more prominent locations and clustering of betting shops in highstreet areas, plus the accumulating evidence – both from personal accounts and observations and from scientific studies – that the controversial but highly profitable fixed odds betting terminals, the FOBTs, had altered the nature of betting shops, making them increasingly dangerous places (see Chapter 1). They were worried about the risks they posed to local people in the form of heavy gambling losses, increasing debt and encouragement to gamble for groups of vulnerable people such as the young and unemployed. They have also been concerned at the possibility of associated public disorder; for example, loitering of street drinkers around betting shops, disorder amongst disgruntled gamblers and vandalising of gambling machines. But they are also anxious, more generally, about the future sustainability of their highstreets, threatened as they are by declining retail mix.

My experience coming out of the Birmingham station is now a common one for anyone familiar with the streets of Britain's towns and cities. The country's one specialised treatment service for people with gambling problems – under the umbrella of the National Health Service but paid for out of funds donated by the gambling industry[1] – is located in a part of London that is typically mixed in terms of the wealth or relative poverty of its inhabitants. Walking the short distance from the nearest underground station, you take a turn at a crossroads on two corners of which are betting shop outlets operated by two of the big betting companies. On one of the two other corners there is a pawnbroker's shop. A few premises after the turn is an amusement arcade with rows of gambling machines visible from the street, and not much further on another betting shop belonging to a third of the big bookmakers.

One of the most important changes introduced by the British 2005 Gambling Act – little publicised and appreciated by the public – was, as already mentioned in Chapter 1, the abolition of the 'demand test' which had previously required that a gambling operator applying for a new licence had to establish that there was a demand for a new venue which was not being met by existing outlets. There now seems to be relatively little that a local authority can do to stop the kind of proliferation of betting shops which greets me now when I enter and leave the Birmingham New Street station or visit colleagues at the National Problem Gambling Clinic in London.

Research on the uneven geographical distribution of gambling outlets is particularly relevant to the issue of community vulnerability. One Australian study analysed electronic gambling machine (EGM) loss data across 150 suburban areas in Melbourne (Rintoul et al., 2013). Consistent with other research, EGM density correlated with area disadvantage: average gambling losses increased regularly across five groups of areas, ranging from least to most socially disadvantaged. In the most disadvantaged fifth, the mean gambling loss per adult was A$849 compared with A$298 in the least disadvantaged. Discussing their findings, the authors say (p 334):

> The vulnerability of disadvantaged communities to EGM related harm is much greater than that of more resilient, socioeconomically advantaged communities. . . . It is therefore likely that the location and density of EGMs . . . intensifies the harm associated with EGM use by concentrating it in areas where existing health and other socioeconomic inequalities are already apparent . . . it appears that current EGM arrangements place a disproportionate burden of cost on the most disadvantaged in the community, thus entrenching and exacerbating inequality. . . . Current EGM regulation appears to be counter to public health efforts to reduce the variance in health distribution.

The first study to be carried out in Britain which examined how EGMs are distributed across the country and how the concentration of such machines relates to social and economic characteristics of the local population produced similar findings (Wardle et al., 2014). The results confirmed the hypothesis that gambling machines are not randomly located but are more heavily concentrated in areas where there are more people in lower status occupations, where a higher proportion of people have relatively low incomes and where there are higher proportions of ethnic minority groups and relatively many under-35s, as well as relatively many aged over 75. EGM venues were found to be more densely concentrated in the main urban areas, regional centres and in coastal towns where there are more 'family entertainment centres' – the arcades where children are allowed to play gambling machines as part of the 'traditional seaside experience'. The general pattern is similar to the Australian one even though the types of machines differ as well as the places in which most are to be found – pubs and clubs in Australia and amusement arcades, betting shops, bingo halls and elsewhere in Britain. In both countries it is the relatively poor who have a higher concentration of gambling opportunities in their areas, who have the shorter average distance to travel to their closest EGM (Pearce *et al.*, 2008), who lose a much higher proportion of their incomes gambling, and from whose communities a greater proportion of their collective wealth is extracted.

The Australian harms study (Langham *et al.*, 2016) listed a number of potential local community harms from gambling, including increased demands on health, welfare and social services and the harmful impact on local businesses due to absenteeism and job turnover and business closures. Others have drawn attention to the costs to a community as a result of other businesses being displaced by a large new gambling facility such as a casino complex (Goodman, 1995) and damage to the environment due, for example, to traffic congestion, crowding and noise (Grinols, 2003). Just as significant, if not more so, however, are less tangible or less immediate changes brought about to the character of an area and the loss of local control over the amenities and nature of a community (Australian Productivity Commission, 1999; McMillen, 2003). In Britain, the main operators of EGMs in betting shops argue that they are innocent of the charge that they deliberately target poorer communities. But it is difficult to accept that a highly savvy industry would be unaware of where profits were most likely to be made and would not make commercial decisions on the basis of that intelligence.

The Australian reviewers make another very important point when they say that commercial gambling is now much more 'disembedded' from local cultures than it once was. At one time it might have been said that gambling was part of or had emerged from aspects of the local culture, but no longer. There are illustrations of this around the world from cultures as contrasting as urban Britain and rural aboriginal Australia. The game of pitch and toss, popular in England until well into the 20th century, can be seen as one example of a culturally consonant form of gambling. Interest in horse racing at the nearest horse-racing track, with intense local support for and backing of local favourites, was another (Clapson, 1992).

In Australia the Yalata Aboriginal community exercised its right to prevent a local non-indigenous business from installing poker machines on their premises on the grounds that gambling on regular card games, officially illegal, was a culturally familiar practice and much less destructive. As the anthropologist Maggie Brady (2004) points out, the people in the community were already poor, and when they gambled at cards the winnings were distributed through the community and no one went hungry; whereas if pokies were introduced the money would leave the community and everyone would go hungry. The important distinction that the community was drawing is between gambling as an understood and locally containable social and cultural practice on the one hand and, on the other hand, externally regulated commercial forms of gambling which are alien and threatening in their nature. As Maggie put it, pokies had now come to be seen as agents of bad rather than good, of regressive rather than progressive taxation, of daylight robbery rather than redistributive justice.

Harms to culture and society

The normalisation of gambling

Much less well developed in the new harms approach to gambling, now emerging in Australia, Britain and elsewhere, are gambling's harms to culture and society more generally. The Australian harms report does refer to 'cultural harm' but appears to see this as a further rippling out of the harm associated with problem gambling from the individual gambler to family and friends and thence to community and culture. The bigger questions of what damage gambling might be doing to a country's cultural fabric and what its proper place should be in 21st century society are going largely unasked. They are arguably the most important questions.

The Australian report does list the normalisation of gambling, however, saying, 'A strong theme within the data was that the normalisation of gambling and the pervasive embedding of gambling in other activities such as sport, was a community level intergenerational harm' (Langham *et al.*, 2016). One way in which citizens are regularly exposed to gambling is through advertising. The ubiquity of gambling advertising, its frequently aggressive tone, and its ethically questionable and continual emphasis on winning, highlighted in Chapter 4, have been widely criticised (Binde, 2009; Derevensky *et al.*, 2010; Thomas *et al.*, 2012). The particular dangers of normalisation of gambling for children and young people might be rated one of the most serious potential harms. The trend towards the increasing alignment of sport with gambling and links between social media and gambling are thought by many to be particularly harmful, especially for young males, the group known to be most at risk from gambling problems (Gainsbury *et al.*, 2015; King *et al.*, 2009; and see Chapters 1 & 4).

The possibility that the normalisation of gambling and its increasing commercialisation, standardisation and globalisation under the influence of large, transnational businesses might itself be harmful sits uneasily with the pronouncements of governments which benefit financially from gambling and have a vested interest in underestimating its harms. The British Government, a major pillar of the *Gambling Establishment*, has portrayed gambling as harmless amusement, a leisure activity like any other such commodity to which the public has a right, hindered by as few restrictions as possible, as a source of cultural and economic enhancement and, above all else, as a good example of ordinary business which ought to be allowed to innovate and flourish (see Chapter 3 and Orford, 2011).

Citizens themselves, on the other hand, tend to be much more conscious of cultural and societal harms. Public attitude surveys in Britain, and in several other countries, have all shown that the weight of public opinion is on the side of believing that gambling is foolish and dangerous; that on balance it is bad rather than good for families, communities and society as a whole; and that it should not be encouraged (Orford *et al.*, 2009; Wardle *et al.*, 2011; and see Chapter 1).

Gambling contributes to inequality

Increasing inequalities of income, wealth and opportunity, even within high income countries, and the association between inequality and physical and mental health, have become of increasing concern and in recent decades have generated a huge volume of social and epidemiological research (Orford, 2008). The role of gambling in contributing to social and health inequalities has until recently attracted little attention, but that has been changing. For example, the UK IPPR (2016) report highlighted the findings that problem gambling, as well as being more common amongst men and amongst younger adults, is more common in those on lower incomes and amongst black and ethnic minority groups in Britain. As they said, problem gambling is helping to entrench and exacerbate socio-economic disadvantage. And the international review by Sulkunen *et al.* (2019) concluded that the least advantaged, already experiencing financial stress, job insecurity and other forms of deprivation, are at the greatest risk of problems with gambling. As a result, gambling-related problems accumulate in the very populations that have the most limited means to face them.

It is often found that higher income individuals and households on average spend more on gambling in absolute terms than poorer individuals and households, but as a proportion of their income the poorer spend more on gambling (Grun & McKeigue, 2000; Castrén *et al.*, 2013). Studies from both Britain (Orford *et al.*, 2010) and Germany (Beckert & Lutter, 2009), found that those in the lowest income quintile were spending an average of 12–14% of their net income on gambling compared to only 2% or less in the highest quintile. The social inequality factor in gambling may be stronger for some forms of gambling, such as lottery participation and EGM gambling, than for others. People may be persuaded by the argument that buying lottery tickets helps to support good causes, but this hides the fact that state lotteries constitute a very regressive form of taxation since revenues are disproportionately collected from low income segments of the population, particularly those receiving social welfare benefits (Sulkunen *et al.*, 2019). Gambling can be seen as, in effect, a form of money transfer from the poor to the more wealthy, encouraged by governments but aggravating inequality. Evidence reviewed by Sulkunen *et al.* supports the charge that government gambling revenues are a form of 'regressive taxation'.

Studies from the USA and New Zealand have suggested that economic downturns may strengthen the relationship between gambling and income inequality. A time-series analysis of over 50 years of US data showed that spending on lotteries was maintained or increased during recessions (Horváth & Paap, 2012). Analysis of New Zealand health survey data from 2008, 2010 and 2012 found that although overall gambling participation had dropped following the financial crisis, households experienced more gambling-related harm in 2012 compared with the earlier years. Residents of more deprived areas were 4.5 times more likely to experience gambling-related problems than those from wealthier neighbourhoods (Tu *et al.*, 2014). In the UK, too, analysis of the adult psychiatric morbidity survey found an association between area deprivation and gambling problems (Carrà *et al.*, 2017), and the same has been found in the USA (Welte *et al.*, 2004).

Various explanations have been put forward to explain why poorer people tend to gamble to their disadvantage. One is that gambling offers to many the only perceived possibility of escaping poverty or being able to purchase otherwise unaffordable consumer goods. The idea of gambling being motivated by the desire to ease financial constraints, if only in a small and temporary way, was supported by the results of a piece of research carried out for the National Lottery Commission in Britain. Women were asked whether they thought the National Lottery was a form of gambling – 88% thought it was – and why they played. The most cited motivation for playing was because of the chance of winning the jackpot. Although giving money to charity was often rated as important, the possibility of winning was much more likely to be rated as *very important*. The most popular way in which women imagined they would spend winnings was to purchase 'treats' for themselves or their families. It was less boredom that women sought to ease, as is sometimes suggested, the report's authors concluded, but more to do with relieving guilt and anxiety, less an escape through the act of gambling itself and more the dream of a jackpot offering opportunity to ease some of the women's everyday concerns about money. The women who took part were often stressed about money and felt guilty because their lack of funds meant they could not provide for their families as they would like to. For example (Casey, 2003, p 255):

> Just to pay off my mortgage and have an easier lifestyle really . . . not to have to scrimp and save up for things all the time you know? . . . Just to make it a bit easier than what it is now, just to get a bit more money really. I'd have that much extra every month. So I wouldn't need to win loads you know?

The Sulkunen *et al.* (2019) international review concludes in no doubt that gambling contributes to inequality and that the more that gambling opportunities are created, the more social inequality is likely to increase.

Gambling's harm to the good life for all

There are still bigger questions to be asked. What contribution might modern commercial gambling – diverse, easily accessible and vigorously promoted with the encouragement of government – be making to a society in which inequality and income insecurity have risen, austerity is promoted politically and personal and family debt has been encouraged? Does gambling increasingly represent one way in which people with reduced prospects and opportunities can maintain hope for a brighter future? Does it aid the further development of a 'risk society' (Beck, 1992) generally, an 'age of chance' (Reith, 1999), or one more accepting of there being 'winners' and 'losers'? Such things are matters for debate. But if there is any truth in such speculations, it could be said that therein might lie the biggest harms of all.

In a democratic country we have representatives whom we rely upon to address the broader issues to do with the kind of world we want to live in. It turns out that there is a large disconnect between what the gambling industry and its government and other supporters – the *Gambling Establishment* – tell us is good for us in the way of more gambling as an entertainment product and the attitudes of the public who are much less welcoming of increased gambling. We need to be asking not just whether gambling is harmful or harmless in rather narrow utilitarian terms but whether more gambling increases the quality of life for us all. In their book, *How Much Is Enough? Money and the Good Life*, dealing with the role of ethics and values in modern life, Skidelsky and Skidelsky (2013) argue that liberalism has been hijacked and has gone terribly wrong: 'liberal thinkers have insisted on public neutrality between rival conceptions of the good. The state . . . should not throw its weight behind this or that ethical outlook'. The modern version of the liberal state, the Skidelskys say, glorifies neutrality and embodies no positive vision of its own. Gambling is a prime case of what they are talking about. Its defence is primarily commercial, and any criticism of it must be justified in utilitarian terms, such as the cost to the state of any crime, lost productivity or the need for health care associated with 'problem gambling'. In an ethically neutral world, our views about whether gambling, widely available and promoted, is consonant or not with family, community and national values – the really important kinds of question – are not on the agenda. Meanwhile there are some obvious beneficiaries of this value neutrality. The neutral state, according to the Skidelskys, 'simply hands power to the guardians of capital to manipulate public taste in their own interests'.

In fact, the British Government, for one, has not been totally successful in stifling discussion of values. In the week following the publication of the report of the Gambling Review Body (2001), on which the Government based the liberalising 2005 Gambling Act, Lord Hattersley, former Deputy Leader of the British Labour Party, wrote (Daily Mail, 2001):

> It seems possible that Britain . . . will become the gambling capital of Europe. . . . The problem now is . . . a gradual and corrosive destruction of

the values on which our society is based. Nobody can be sure the casinos will not become easy territory for drug pushers, but we can be certain that, once the international gamblers move in, they will be fertile ground for men who want to take money from people who cannot afford it. . . . We have to ask, is it worth it?

Conclusion

In this chapter I have taken the new 'harms approach' to gambling, looking broadly at the public health, social and community harms of gambling. It has been argued that the acceptance of gambling in its present forms as a normal part of modern society threatens that society's health and well-being in a number of ways: by adversely affecting ill-health, homelessness and crime statistics, diminishing the vibrancy of town centres, contributing to inequality and adding to the risks faced by the young. In the process it may be a contributor to the undermining of some of the values which a society holds most dear.

The costs for individuals with gambling problems and for their families remain, I believe, the deepest and most significant harms associated with gambling. Most of those costs are emotional and personal and almost impossible for economists to quantify, which is perhaps why they tend to be underappreciated and over-looked. The health consequences of problem gambling are mainly in the area of mental health, which is the poor relation of physical health and the more difficult to count. The very word 'costs' implies that we should be endeavouring to put a price on the impact of problem gambling on health and happiness. But how can you put a cost on the experience of being so overwhelmed by a gambling habit that your thoughts turn to the possibility of suicide, or on the experience of living daily with the uncertainty of whether your partner is gambling away your family's security and hopes, or on a child's experience of repeatedly being let down by a parent who is more attentive to gambling online than to you?

It requires political leadership to get a grip on the evidence of gambling's harms to individuals, families, communities and society. In the next chapter I shall argue that the *Gambling Establishment*, far from providing that leadership, has in fact taken a biased and self-serving approach to the evidence.

Notes

1 A second such clinic has now opened in the north of England and NHS funding for the clinics has, I understand, now been agreed.

8

HOW THE GAMBLING ESTABLISHMENT HAS USED EVIDENCE TO SUPPORT ITS POSITION

There is no simple relationship between research and policy

Despite the evidence of a growing backlash against unrestrained growth of modern commercial gambling, reform is strongly resisted by the gambling-providing industry and its allies inside and outside government. An argument which is often forwarded in an effort to mollify calls for reform is the appeal for more research: only if research shows clear evidence of harm caused by a particular type or mode of gambling or the way it is promoted should the business of providing gambling be restrained, it is argued.

There is a fundamental point that needs to be made about gambling research, as about much policy research, and it is one that is either misunderstood, completely overlooked or deliberately forgotten by the *Gambling Establishment*. This is the point that there is no simple relationship between research and policy. The elementary assumption has been that policymakers have a problem they need to solve, that they then use research findings or commission new research to fill the gap in knowledge, and that they then make decisions based on the results. For some time now this understanding of the way research and policy relate to one another – variously referred to as the linear, rational or purist model – has been seriously challenged in health and social policy circles (Glasby, 2011). It is now widely recognised that the relationship between research and policy is much more complex, messier, even 'disorderly', as one writer put it. The simple model has particular difficulty fitting the reality of what goes on in highly politicised or controversial areas. In practice, it is often a mixture of 'evidence-based policy' and 'policy-based evidence'. Other terms that have been appearing include 'evidence-informed policy' and 'evidence-inspired policy'. It is no accident that in Britain we used to have a Centre for Evidence-based Policy but now we have a Centre for Evidence *and* Policy.

The gambling evidence–policy link is a clear example of this, but it is certainly not alone. The way research evidence is used, or not used as the case may be, to influence drugs policy is another obvious example. It is interesting to note in passing how very different are the officially sanctioned positions on the harms associated with an illegal market for drugs and the legalised market for gambling. In the former case the dominant discourse, and preferred forms of evidence, focus on the dangers of the 'product', such as whether the harmfulness of cannabis is sufficient to place it in a higher harm category for legal purposes. When it comes to gambling, on the other hand, Establishment discourse has emphasised the legitimacy and harmlessness of the product and the duty of the consumer to consume it responsibly, even denying that any one form of the product is any more dangerous than another.

Values, which have been downplayed in gambling policy as we saw in the previous chapter, come into the picture here too (Monaghan, 2011). UK Governments, notably New Labour, promised more Government accountability linked to the idea of replacing political values with objective scientific evidence in policy-making – framed by politicians as 'value-free policy'. A principal criticism of evidence-based policy has been that there is a danger of removing political values from policy debates – a process of 'depoliticisation'. By suggesting that policy decisions should be value-free and made on the basis of objective evidence, it might appear to leave out of consideration the need to make any judgements about what constitutes 'the good society' and what kind of evidence is prioritised. In the drugs case, amongst the drug policy 'establishment' and 'critical friends' of the Government there was a great emphasis on the nature of substances themselves in terms of scientifically assessing their risks and the importance of maintaining a hierarchy of drugs in terms of their harms. However, many interest groups thought the policy debate was too narrow, focussing on individual harm, particularly physical harm, neglecting mental, intellectual, social, emotional, spiritual and environmental harm, the harmful effects on others such as family and friends, and the harm that occurs before addiction develops, such as any harm from intoxication. Others believed that decision-makers were failing to show an appreciation of the way in which drug prohibition contributes to problems and how the futility of prohibition is left out of the decision-making process. Any such suggestion of the need for evidence related to wider issues such as the success or otherwise of prohibition, was easily dismissed by the establishment as being 'ideologically driven and speculative'. In other words, evidence utilisation involves issues of power.

There is now recognition that policy-making is in reality more piecemeal or 'muddled through' than the simple model of evidence-based policy would suggest (Russell & Greenhalgh, 2011). One view is that new research is unlikely to have a bearing on predetermined positions allied to various interests and ideologies. A more positive view of how evidence influences policy, sometimes termed the 'enlightenment model', sees the process as one of 'indirect diffusion' whereby an entire body of research or evidence, accumulating over time, sensitises policy-makers to new issues. A more 'interactive' model of what goes on suggests that research is not the only factor influencing decision-making, that policymakers engage in consultations with a range of stakeholders, eventually moving towards a policy response: particularly in politicised areas, 'concepts and therefore knowledge are inherently contested and meaning emerges from negotiation and dialogue between relevant constituents'.

Criticisms of the way in which 'evidence' is being produced and used in the modern gambling field

How the way gambling research is funded has failed to guarantee independence

All of which is extremely pertinent to gambling policy and how evidence is produced and used in the modern liberalised era. In March 2014 a day conference was held at Goldsmiths, University of London, to launch an important report which addressed the controversial issue of how gambling research is produced. The title of the report was, *Fair Game: Producing Gambling Research. The Goldsmiths Report.* It was based on interviews with more than 100 gambling researchers, policymakers and industry members, over half from the UK, with others from elsewhere in Europe, Hong Kong, Macau, Australia and North America. The conclusions do not make for comfortable reading. There was much here about lack of research funding, the comparatively low status of gambling research, absence of cross-fertilisation between gambling studies and related fields, and difficulties in accessing data. The biggest theme, however, was the dependence of gambling research on industry support, a lack of transparency about this, and a poor understanding in the field about conflicts of interest. As the report put it (Cassidy *et al.*, 2013, p 9),

> The interests of funders are reproduced in diverse ways, including in the questions that are prioritised, . . . the ways in which applications are assessed and the ways in which research is disseminated. Voluntary contributions . . . are conceptualised as gifts. . . . This allows the industry to maintain a sense of ownership over research.

In addition to the report's authors, there were others who spoke at the conference and provided valuable background to the report. One was Peter Adams from the University of Auckland, New Zealand, whom we met earlier (in Chapter 3 and other chapters). Perhaps more than anyone else, he has sought, in his writing (e.g. Adams, 2008, 2016) and speaking, to question the whole framework of ideas which govern gambling policy and to expose the ways in which Big Gambling's power is exercised. He spoke about the way in which life in his country has been 'infiltrated' by gambling and how community groups had become dependent on gambling income. He spoke of the need for researchers and others to consider the extent to which taking money jeopardises one's ethical position, depending upon such factors as the extent to which the purposes of the organisations giving and receiving funds are similar or different, the extent and nature of their links, and the type and degree of harm caused by the product in question. He concluded with a call for a new sub-discipline of gambling studies – one that focuses on the industry and its activities.

In a telling comment, Robin Room (2016), a highly respected and well-travelled addiction researcher, says, 'In countries which I know well the gambling field is unusual in the high proportion of its funding which comes from agencies or interests with a vested interest in the gambling market'. In their article calling for 'clear principles . . . for integrity in gambling research', Peter Adams and his Australian colleague Charles Livingstone (2016, p 6) say, correctly in my experience,

> Existing research frequently lacks quality and diversity, and focuses too often on peripheral topics that are acceptable to industry-influenced panels and research application processes. Much of it presents science as an uncomplicated fact-finding exercise, with little consideration for the political economy of knowledge. The existing weak knowledge base enables . . . a kind of strategic inertia, citing a lack of evidence, at the same time as they tell critics of gambling to 'wait and see' what a particular piece of research finds . . . the distinction between industry and academia is blurred.

In his book *Moral Jeopardy: Risks of Accepting Money from the Alcohol, Tobacco and Gambling Industries*, Adams (2016) refers specifically to three prolific gambling researchers based in the three continents that produce the large bulk of gambling research, each of whom has been comfortable receiving money from and working with the gambling industry and each of whom has been criticised for so doing. The criticism is not that they have failed to do good research. In fact, each has led active research teams and contributed greatly to an emerging field over a good many years, and I have leant on their findings at several points in this book. Why I and others have been critical of the model which they have set of accepting industry funding is, rather, because of how the field as a whole is distorted in industry-supporting ways by such heavy reliance on such funding.

One of the three is Alex Blaszczynski, an author of the influential Reno Model of gambling problems, which was mentioned in Chapter 3 as an oft-quoted exposition of academic views on gambling policy which are relatively conservative, industry-supporting ones. He is described by Adams as 'Australia's leading expert on gambling. . . [who has] openly admitted . . . he has accepted [large amounts of] funding directly from gambling-industry sources . . . who episodically speaks in favour of industry interests' (p 104).

The second is Howard Shaffer, affiliated to Harvard Medical School in the USA. Adams details the relationship between the trade body, the American Gambling Association (AGA), the National Center for Responsible Gaming (NCRG), and Harvard's Institute for Research on Gambling (IRG), as a good example of one of the main ways in which industry-researcher links are 'ethically sanitised'.

This involves apparent decoupling of the links by passing the financial support through at least one and often several intermediaries, giving the impression of independence from gambling profits and obscuring ethical doubts. Another internationally prominent addiction researcher and writer, Tom Babor (2016), thinks the AGA/NCRG/IRG case provides a good example of how the 'so-called firewall established by gambling industry sources to limit the influence of industry funding on scientific research . . . fails to prevent important conflicts of interest'.

Adams and the Goldsmiths group are not alone in drawing attention to the thoroughly unsatisfactory state of affairs that exists regarding gambling research. A report from the USA entitled *The Gambling Threat to National and Homeland Security* (Kindt, 2012) is a weighty tome unlikely to be read by anyone other than those with an interest in who said what, when, on the subject inside and outside Congress in the USA in the previous few years. A number of law and business academics at the University of Illinois played a part in this compilation of documents, a primary goal of which was to present facts which would help to correct 'alleged misinformation disseminated by Big Gambling'. Severely criticised is the pro-gambling lobby headed by the AGA, the Harvard IRG, The Boyd Law School at the University of Nevada, Las Vegas, and journals such as the *Gaming Law Review* and the *Journal of Gambling Studies* which the report says were dominated, at least for a time, by pro-gambling interests.

The third prominent gambling researcher Adams mentions is Mark Griffiths of the International Gaming Research Unit at Nottingham Trent University in England. He has done a great deal of good work in the gambling field, and I have on occasions worked with him myself. His acceptance of industry support is symptomatic of the situation regarding the funding of research, prevention and treatment in Britain, which is very unsatisfactory. Funding dedicated to gambling is on a small scale and comes almost entirely directly from the gambling industry. The British research funding chain, though shorter than in the Harvard case, is similar. It involves an industry levy, still only voluntary at the time of writing, passed to the self-acknowledged industry-led body, the Responsible Gambling Trust (RGT), now GambleAware but still heavily influenced by the industry despite its rebranding and change of name, which then decides how to allocate those funds for research (and for treatment and prevention).

This arrangement is at the least highly controversial and at worst a cause for ridicule nationally and internationally. Without a national structure for research and for treatment and prevention which is independent of the powerful provider industry, conflicts of interests are endemic, the field is treated as tarnished by much of the academic community and there is evidence that top researchers are being attracted to other countries.

Some of the necessary independence should be ensured in Britain by the Responsible Gambling Strategy Board (RGSB, recently renamed as the Advisory Board for Safer Gambling), but Adams thinks otherwise. In fact he cites the RGSB as an example of another 'sanitizing practice', the setting up of a supposedly independent panel of experts which advises Government on, amongst other things, what should be research priorities. He points out the many opportunities that exist to influence the membership of such panels to ensure they are not too threatening of industry interests; and they are often advisory only, with final decisions made elsewhere. In the RGSB case, because of the Gambling Commission-GambleAware-RGSB structure, the RGSB, now ABSG, is not an independent advisory body to Government but rather an integral part of the Establishment. Its terms of reference require it to work closely with the Gambling Commission and with GambleAware. For example, its recommendations are expected to be put into effect by GambleAware which will commission research (as well as *education* and treatment), sometimes putting out calls for research bids in conjunction with the Gambling Commission.

RGSB renewed its research strategy every four years. Its lack of true independence was clear from its strategy for 2016 to 2019. Disappointing was the marginalisation of prevention in comparison with treatment and the tendency to equate prevention with education, both things that have also been notable in Government and Gambling Commission statements in recent years. Reliance was inappropriately placed on RGT/GambleAware and the industry to take responsibility for building British research capacity. Nor were the large stakeholder group of families and others affected by someone else's gambling mentioned other than in a rather general and unspecified way.

How the content of research is influenced

More is understood now about how conflicts of interest affect the results of research. Much has been learned from tobacco research and also from pharmaceutical research. An important conclusion is that industry-funded research does tend to result in findings skewed towards industry interests. This is not for the most part because the research is conducted badly or inappropriately, although that can also happen, but because of what happens at either end of the process: in the choice of topics to research in the first place and at the end in how results are reported and especially what finds its way into summaries and conclusions. All early researchers making their first forays into academic publishing are advised to make sure that the abstract or summary that appears at the beginning of the paper is accurate because that is what most people will see. Indeed, most people will never get beyond the abstract, particularly now that electronic searches usually give open access to abstracts only. Longer reports for other purposes, often of greater immediate policy impact, are usually required to start with an 'executive summary', and those who want to influence busy government ministers are usually advised to keep what they say short and to the point. Companies that directly commission research or do so indirectly, 'are then in a position to choose how . . . data is reported, what slant it gets, who receives a copy of the reports and what is emphasized – or, more importantly, what is de-emphasized' (Adams, 2016).

Natasha Schüll (2012), in her book *Addiction by Design*, already cited in Chapter 5, is also critical of what she sees as the 'strong industrial–academic alliance [that] had formed around the understanding of gambling addiction as a discrete disease entity rooted in individual predisposition' and the conflicts of interests involved. Of the NCRG, which had funded most of the gambling addiction research in the USA, she said it 'fund[s] virtually no research on the industry's products and the role they might play in problem gambling . . . the lion's share of NCRG monies support investigations into the genetic, neuroscientific, and psychological determinants of the addiction'. In fact, much of her excellent book can be seen as an effort to redress that lopsided focus by redirecting attention to the design of modern gambling machines themselves. As she says, 'the story of "problem gambling" is not just a story of problem gamblers; it is also a story of problem machines, problem environments, and problem business practices'. Adams (2016, p 124) makes the same point in his book when he says,

> as a consequence of industry influence, gambling research is dominated by "research of convenience", where the emphasis is on tracking problems for individual consumers rather than looking upstream at determinants such as gambling environments and machine design.

This controversy will continue, dividing the research community in the process. Australian academic Martin Young (2013) is another who has criticised the way in which the academic community has bolstered Establishment thinking and interests by focussing so much of their attention on problem or pathological gambling, diverting attention in the process from gambling products, the activities of the gambling industry and wider harms to communities and society. His paper was immediately followed by a published commentary by two leading gambling researchers from Harvard Medical School (Shaffer & LaPlante, 2013). We have already noted in Chapter 5 how the Harvard group wrongly interpreted the skewed distribution findings from their study of online gamblers in a way that supports the industry discourse about problem gambling by emphasising the relatively moderate gambling activity of most players. In their commentary on Young's paper, they now used familiar industry rhetorical arguments such as: the absence of convincing evidence of a causal association between problem gambling prevalence and the growth of the gambling industry; and the harsh economic conditions the gambling industry was now facing.

As Young stated in a reply to their commentary, their argument was a misunderstanding of the critical position he was taking towards the dominance of a particular way of doing science in the gambling field. He and I are in agreement about this. The *Gambling Establishment* has told us how we should be thinking about gambling and is dictating the research agenda. As Young said about the Harvard response to his commentary, 'it is an attempt to privilege one form of understanding and claim to knowledge over another . . . to discredit arguments outside of its own frame of reference'.

A case in point: How British research on high-powered gambling machines was hijacked by the gambling-providing industry

The situation we have in Britain when it comes to gambling research and policy is as good an example as you could wish for of the messiness of the research–policy relationship. It is one I have been very critical of – see the Gambling Watch UK website. The so-called 'gambling machines research' project illustrated the problem. In November 2012, following publicity about the harms believed to be associated with the British variety of modern, technologically sophisticated, fast and high-powered gambling machines – the Fixed Odds Betting Terminals, or FOBTs – the Responsible Gambling Trust (RGT) announced a half-million pound research programme about those types of EGMs.

Or at least everyone thought it was going to be about the machines. To be more accurate, it turned out to be a research programme about people who play such machines. The Chief Executive of RGT said in the announcement that there is a 'lack of robust evidence about how people play on these machines and what helps people to stay in control and play responsibly'. That focus on players' behaviour and their failure to behave responsibly is consistent with *Gambling Establishment* discourse and with its general approach to preventing gambling harm. It is also exactly what we would expect from a body which was in the lap of an industry on the defensive after two highly critical British television programmes that year (Channel 4 *Dispatches* in August, and BBC1 *Panorama* in November) and the efforts of an increasingly successful campaign (the Campaign for Fairer Gambling) against the siting of such high-stake gambling machines – or as the RGT announcement called them, 'gaming machines' – in highstreet betting shops. Unlike a proper public health programme of research, which would also look at the danger to which people are exposed and the environment in which exposure takes place, it seemed this programme of research would only be looking at the behaviour of the people exposed to the danger.

It was stressed in the announcement that the industry would collaborate fully in the research. This was a clever move on the industry's part, provided of course that the research did not focus too closely on the addictive nature of the machines themselves, the profits they were making at the expense of problem gamblers, or the story of how such machines had been allowed in betting shops without a proper social and health impact assessment. The announcement made it look as if the industry was itself acting responsibly, unlike the people who become casualties of their dangerous products. It also had the effect of disarming criticism, hiding behind the 'more research is needed' argument, assuming that high-stake machines were here to stay and kicking into the long grass any consideration of profit-threatening moves, such as whether FOBTs should be made safer by bringing the maximum stake size into line with other gambling machines or by banning them from highstreet betting shops altogether.

The first reports of the research were presented to an audience largely consisting of industry representatives at a conference held in London in December 2014.

This was an important occasion not least because those who had been arguing for something significant to be done about FOBTs in betting shops were told that no policy decisions would be taken until this research had reported. The suspicion that the research would follow the industry lead in focussing on problem play and problem players rather than on problem products was immediately confirmed. It was repeatedly stated in the reports and during discussion at the conference that the main purpose of the programme was 'to identify problem gamblers and harmful patterns of play'.

Central to this industry-funded research was betting transaction data provided by the five big British bookmaking companies (Wardle, 2014). This was lauded by RGT as being the first of its kind in Britain, as being the largest set of such data yet assembled anywhere in the world and as demonstrating industry goodwill and willingness to collaborate. The size of the database was indeed huge – more than 6.7 billion bets placed in over 32,000 gambling machines in over 8,000 betting shops! The *Gambling Establishment* is taking a lot of interest in these kinds of data and is putting a lot of faith in the prospect of thereby unlocking the secrets of how people gamble and why some don't gamble 'responsibly'.

A survey of those holding loyalty cards with three of the big betting companies enabled information about individuals to be linked to the betting transactional data. A particular aim was to determine what parameters of machine play best predicted whether someone had a score on the Problem Gambling Severity Index indicating a gambling problem. The report's authors claimed that they had shown they could predict problem gambling and that there was therefore 'a bright future for behavioural analytics' in the area of social responsibility and gambling. This was really over-optimistic and smacked of special pleading. Of course, no one expects perfect prediction, but the results were hardly impressive since they showed, for example, that 50% of problem gamblers could be identified but only at a cost of a false-positive rate of 25% amongst the larger group of non-problem gamblers. This represents an unacceptably high false-positive rate. In other words, at even a modest level of sensitivity, specificity was unacceptably low.

This programme of research, although there was much about it which was very interesting, is a good example of how the gambling research agenda has been hijacked by the gambling industry and those who have been taken in by their overall view of things. One obvious indication of this was the makeup of the organisations that collaborated to sponsor, oversee and carry out the research. In an attempt to provide some independence from the industry, a Machines Research Oversight Panel was set up. Its well-chosen chair was none other than Alex Blaszc-zynski, one of the world's leading industry-supported academics (see above). In a speech made on his behalf at the conference, it was stated that, despite industry support for the research programme, it did seem that the work had been independently carried out (Delfabbro, 2014). This is really to miss the point. The research was probably carried out, and mostly reported, without direct influence by the industry. The real point is that the research required the collaboration of the industry which provided access to much of the data, and the very nature of the research and the questions being asked were part of a whole framework of ideas about 'responsible gambling' which is industry-friendly and not too industry-challenging. One then has to ask about members of the collaborating research team. The well-known British social research organisation NatCen has an excellent record of carrying out independent research and is generally considered to be above reproach. One of the other research partners, however, was an organisation called Featurespace, which has a history of working with the gambling industry, has contracts with the industry and has gambling industry representation on its board. Even before the conference they had been accused of drawing unwarranted, industry-favourable, conclusions in a press release and tweets, and that part of the report led by Featurespace displayed an obvious bias (Excell & Bobashev, 2014). It repeatedly referred to 'a small number of extreme values', 'a small number of significant outliers', the majority of players exhibiting 'minimal values' and most variables following an exponential curve so 'large values . . . are very rare'. This is a coded way of saying: Look how moderate almost all machine play is and how rare is immoderate or irresponsible gambling! In actual fact, the results provided ample evidence of the large amounts of money that many people were losing in quite short periods of time. For example, they showed that it is not at all uncommon for players to be losing over £100 in little more than half an hour (see the discussion in Chapter 5 about the importance of understanding skewed frequency distribution curves).

The front cover of the printed programme for the conference day bore the Featurespace logo alongside logos for IGT, Rank, and Joelson Wilson, respectively 'the industry's leading manufacturer of gaming machines', owners of a large casino chain, and a law firm that 'advises remote gambling operators and suppliers, acting for spread-betting companies, online casinos and major betting websites'.

The likely conclusions that the industry and their supporters would draw from this programme of research came out in the final panel discussion at the conference. A remark made by a senior officer of the Gambling Commission sums up the whole problem with the way the research programme had been set up by saying that the takeout message was that 'we should be looking at people not the product'. That seems to be strange coming from the body that is charged with regulating the industry. The Chief Executive of one of the very biggest betting companies, prominent in Britain and very active elsewhere, was clearer still in concluding that, 'it's not the product'. The keyword for him, to summarise the research findings, was 'complex' – very convenient of course for an industry making huge profits out of a dangerous activity. The Featurespace report opined, 'The focus should shift away from regulating particular parameters, such as stake size, but take a balanced rounded approach which considers the player, the product and the environment', an apparently uncontentious statement but a clear reference nevertheless to the debate about the very high stakes on FOBT machines. The Oversight Panel chair made essentially the same point at the end of his written introduction:

at this stage, it would be inadvisable to rush policies on the basis of these foundational studies . . . more would be achieved by a strategic approach compared to fragmented, disjointed and potentially costly policies that fail to achieve their objective.

The message from the *Gambling Establishment* was clear – the research shows how complicated everything is, and our reading of the research allows us to deflect the demands we have been hearing that high-stake, FOBT-type gambling machines are dangerous and should be modified or taken out of betting shops.

What we have here with this particular British case is a perfect example of the way in which research can be used – hijacked is my preferred word for it – to support a powerful Establishment position. This is done by using existing evidence selectively, loading advisory committees, commissioning research in such a way that it is less likely to pose Establishment-challenging questions or come up with results that are detrimental to the established policy direction, choosing ways of publicising results other than via proper peer-reviewed publication, and providing a particular interpretation of findings. These mechanisms relate to the way power exerts its influence on the relationship between evidence and policy-making. They are familiar to those who have observed how research in the health and social sciences can be used in controversial areas. They were all on show in the gambling machines research. Fortunately, in 2018, as described in Chapter 1, events overtook the industry and its supporters in the form of concerted pressure for reform, resulting in belated Government agreement to act to drastically reduce maximum FOBT stake size.

A second case in point: the use of evidence to resist calls for a 9.00 pm TV gambling advertising watershed

A second example of the way in which evidence is being called upon in a selective and misleading way is to do with gambling advertising. One of the things contributors to the Gambling Watch UK website express repeatedly is their annoyance and alarm at the amount of gambling advertising they have had to put up with since the 2005 Gambling Act came fully into operation in Britain in 2007. Parents are especially alarmed at the amount of such advertising their children are exposed to. It is an accepted principle, in the case of material which is generally agreed children should be protected from seeing on television, that containing violence or sex for example, that 9.00 pm is an appropriate 'watershed', before which such material should not be shown. In my discussions with the Gambling Commission, it has acknowledged that the decision to allow live sports gambling advertising before the watershed was not based on any evidence that it would not be harmful but was, rather, a trade-off with the industry agreed at the time that the 2005 Gambling Act was being formulated.

It seems that no evidence was required when the decision was made to allow pre-watershed advertising, whereas now rigorous evidence would be required of harm in order to have it banned as parents and others would like. This was made quite clear in a report from the Committee of Advertising Practice and the Broadcast Committee of Advertising Practice (CAP & BCAP, 2015). Most of the report, supposedly about evidence relevant to the issue, was actually not about that at all but consisted instead of a lengthy background explanation of what CAP and BCAP and the ASA (Advertising Standards Authority) do and what their rules and codes cover. When it finally got on to the subject of evidence, the report acknowledged that the amount of gambling advertising had increased enormously since 2005. There were then 90,000 spot adverts, mostly TV adverts, a figure that had risen to 1.4 million in 2012. Those figures equate to 5.8 billion person 'impacts' or viewings in 2005, rising to 30 billion in 2012. That is 630 per adult viewer. The figures for 4-to-15-year-olds were 0.5 billion impacts in 2005, rising to 1.8 billion in 2012 (see also Chapter 4).

The report drew on two reviews: one general, specially commissioned, review by Swedish academic Per Binde (2014), whom we first met in Chapter 4, and a second which focussed specifically on children and young people (Monaghan *et al.*, 2008), as well as gambling and health surveys. Otherwise, it relied a lot on what they were told by the Gambling Commission. The general conclusion was that the present rules were more or less in the right place. On the specific issue of pre-watershed advertising, the report concluded that there was no convincing evidence that this was harmful, and therefore no change was required.

In the process of reaching these conclusions, the familiar Establishment device of minimising the recognition of harm was much in evidence. For example, the general consensus, the report said, was that advertising has little causal role in producing harm except possibly in the case of encouraging further gambling by people who already have gambling problems – a group referred to, in familiar Establishment language, as a 'small minority'. When it came to children and young people, they also referred to the proportion who have gambling problems as 'relatively small'. Also on display was the tactic of picking those bits of evidence which seem to fit with current policy. The report acknowledged that there was some evidence of the effect of gambling advertising on young people, for example on their attitudes. But drawing on work on food advertising particularly, it concluded that there is only a modest direct effect of gambling advertising on children and young people. It was emphasised that, in any case, 55% of TV gambling adverts were shown after 9.00 pm and less than 10% (excluding lotteries and scratch cards) between 5.00 pm and 9.00 pm. Most pre-9.00 pm advertising, they said, was for lotteries and scratch cards or bingo, and children saw on average less than one sports or casino gaming advert per week.

In conclusion, 'CAP and BCAP do not consider that there are grounds to support the view that gambling advertising is a significant contributory factor to underage participation'. Never mind that this is a highly contentious conclusion and that many experts who have looked at this closely come to a different view, as we noted in Chapter 4. The report's complacency was summed up in their conclusion that the existing rules met a key objective of the 2005 Gambling Act – to protect children and young people from harm.

There are places in the report where the real issues that concern the public are touched on. A particular focus of complaints to the ASA about gambling advertisements – complaints were up fourfold since 2005 – had been about 'free bets' and also 'bet now' messages. But a lot were about 'advertising generally'. This links to what Binde recognised as the issue of societal values or what he called the 'moral dimension', including concern that advertising is contributing to the normalisation of gambling. But as the report so aptly put it, 'a degree of "normalisation" was envisaged as an acceptable consequence of the [2005] Act by Parliament at the time'. The stimulation of demand was allowed for the first time, and there was greater freedom to advertise. Therefore in their view the issue was not whether normalisation was occurring since it was virtually written into the law when it was formulated. In any case, in the report's opinion, advertising brings 'benefit to consumers in informing them of opportunities'.

There was also a hint of something more fundamental in a section of the report on possible general consumer harm. It referred here specifically to Binde's conclusion that gambling advertisements can be deceptive because they give a misleading impression of the likelihood of winning (see Chapter 4). But the report did not consider that this was something they should act on. For one thing, they thought that always providing information about the odds of winning would be problematic. That is certainly true (see Chapter 5), but not only for the practical and logistical reasons which they probably had in mind. Requiring that the operators of modern forms of gambling, such as the new breeds of gambling machines, display the real odds of winning would threaten the very basis of the profit-making enterprise. But more importantly, the report's understanding of deception was a narrow one. For example, it was thought that advertising free bets would be contrary to the rules only if, for example, important 'terms and conditions' were not specified. But in actual fact the current rule on the matter is sufficiently broad to question exactly the kind of misleading impression about winning which Binde (2009; and see Chapter 4) had exposed in his earlier work. The existing rule would allow complaints to be upheld if it was thought that consumers would be encouraged 'to make an economic decision that they would not otherwise have taken if, for instance, additional information was presented'. It is not difficult to see how many gambling advertisements, which do not specify the actual odds of winning, could be seen to fall foul of that ruling.

It is abundantly clear that CAP and BCAP were effectively operating as loyal elements of the *Gambling Establishment*. Along with others who it was thought might have a special interest in the matter, I was asked to comment on their report. I declined to do so because it was clear that people were being asked to comment on how the present rules were being interpreted and not on the rules themselves. In fact, about the consultation process it was explicitly stated that, 'This process is not an appropriate forum in which to consider calls for more fundamental regulatory change'. But the present framework of rules, which we were told was not to be challenged, was erected some years ago through a process in which industry lobbying and short-sighted economic considerations played the large part. Public concerns and broader questions of values and the good of society played little role. So, once in place, the Establishment framework sets the rules about 'evidence'.

Actually, the main point made by the relevant academic reviews, a point downplayed in the CAP/BCAP report, was that really there is not much firm evidence at all on the subject of advertising and gambling, and more research is needed. But now that the public is bombarded with gambling advertising, including pre-watershed advertising, the requirement for evidence is firmly biased in the direction of the status quo. The evidence-based policy argument, to which Government is so attached and to which the *Gambling Establishment* constantly appeals, runs in one direction. If you think there is too much gambling advertising or that children and young people are harmed by watching gambling advertisements early in the evening, show us the evidence that this is harmful – 'harm' always being defined in fairly narrow terms. We do not need to show you evidence that the public likes such advertising or that it is safe.

Conclusion

In this chapter I have tried to show how the process of gathering evidence about gambling and the harm that it may be doing is being unduly influenced, all along the way from deciding what questions should be asked to interpreting existing evidence and drawing conclusions for policy, by the gambling-providing industry and its supporters. I have used two British examples to illustrate what I mean. I have made the point that I am not alone in holding this view. Furthermore, this is not an extreme opinion since it fits with conclusions reached by many who have looked at the tortuous ways in which evidence is used, misused or ignored in the process of supporting or challenging social policy in areas well beyond gambling.

The conclusions of this chapter play an important role in the book's general argument. The *Gambling Establishment* is a powerful collective. At its core sits the gambling-providing industry, particularly the large, internationally active companies whose profits depend upon newly developed, dangerous ways of helping people part with their money. But around that core lie others who either keenly support that industry or who, more commonly, are obliged to support it because their jobs, income or careers depend on supporting it. Many may be unaware that they are supporting it. But they are supporting it by openly or tacitly lending their weight in support of a particular way of interpreting facts and opinions on the subject. They may not all be powerful players in themselves, but collectively they are helping to impose on us all a way of thinking and understanding about gambling and along with it an acceptance of more, and more dangerous, gambling. The way in which the *Gambling Establishment*'s power is used to influence the research process is part of that.

9

RESISTING THE POWER OF THE GAMBLING ESTABLISHMENT

A manifesto for change

In this chapter, I outline a number of proposals for the way forward. The proposals that follow are designed with the British gambling context in mind. However, it is evident that the issues my country faces, although it certainly has its peculiarities when it comes to gambling, are much the same ones being confronted around the world. My recommendations – a manifesto for gambling regulation in the 2020s and 2030s if you like – may therefore have relevance elsewhere. My proposals for change are summarised in brief in Table 9.1.

Getting the basics right: the need for new thinking, new legislation, new strategy

As recent developments, outlined in Chapter 1, have shown, it is becoming increasingly clear that Britain, for one, made a big mistake when it passed the 2005 Gambling Act. The Act is turning out to be sufficiently flawed that a completely new Act based on different principles is now needed. The Labour Party (2017), responsible for the 2005 Act when it was then in power, in order to put things right, has now called for this. A new Act will need not simply to make changes to the details of how gambling is commercially provided – details such as the maximum stake allowed on certain categories of EGMs or the permitted hours for TV advertisements, important though such details are – but also to go back to basics and get the fundamentals right. First and foremost, it will need a rethink about the ideology which has dominated official thinking about gambling regulation: the Establishment discourse about gambling will need to change. Also to be rethought will be the roles of Government and the industry in gambling policy formation and the funding of gambling harm prevention, treatment and research. The industry must step back, and Government must step forward. A National Government Strategy for Gambling will be required with changes to where within Government responsibility lies.

TABLE 9.1 A manifesto for how gambling should be better managed in Britain (and elsewhere) in the 2020s and 2030s

The basics rethought: how we view gambling and the role of Government and the industry	Replacement of the ordinary business/responsible gambling ideology with an alternative dangerous consumption/public health perspective
	A proper national strategy for gambling produced by Government
	Gambling seen in Government as a cross-department issue with the Health Ministry playing a leading role
	Gambling harm prevention, treatment and research (PT&R) funded out of general taxation, with gambling tax increased to bring Britain into line with other countries
	The funding of gambling harm PT&R administered by a new body such as a National Gambling Council or Institute completely independent of the industry or regulator
	Britain to be a major contributor to a global framework of principles for gambling regulation
The issue of gambling advertising reconsidered, with the protection of children and young people as a primary consideration	A proper pre-watershed ban on television advertising, including the pre-match period
	Removal of all gambling advertising visible during sporting fixtures popular with children and young people
	Gambling company sponsorship of football and other sporting clubs banned, as in a number of countries
	The introduction of children to gambling through social media examined and appropriate measures taken
	Advertising standards/codes reconsidered from scratch
Harm-reduction policies reconsidered, shifting the emphasis away from reliance on ineffective forms of HR such as education and tracking and identifying problem players towards HR measures of sufficient scope and magnitude which render gambling products less dangerous	A minimum age of 18 years for all gambling, including the National Lottery and low-stake/low-prize EGMs, with continued improvement in age verification
	Any proposed new form of gambling, mode or type of venue subject to a full social, health and economic impact assessment
	Clearer adherence to the principle of preventing ambient gambling
	Reconsider local option to allow, limit or ban certain forms of gambling
	Further improvement in comprehensive self-exclusion schemes
	Some combination of absolute and mandatory-self-chosen loss- and time-limit setting
	Support for methods that limit the ease or immediacy of accessing funds for gambling
	Removal of gambling design features which encourage faulty cognitions and increase game intensity, such as large stake and prize sizes, sound and visual effects, near misses, and losses disguised as wins
	Smoking and alcohol use in gambling venues prohibited

(Continued)

TABLE 9.1 (Continued)

A proper comprehensive system of treatment for people with gambling problems and help for their families	The availability of treatment for gambling problems increased, ranging from a small number of regional specialist centres and community residential facilities to brief, early interventions, telephone helplines and online support; NHS involvement increased
	Consciousness about gambling problems improved among staff of primary health care, mental health, social service, debt, law enforcement, and homelessness services, as well as educational and other services for children and young people
	The volume and quality of gambling treatment research increased
	Provision made for affected family members to play a role in treatment and to receive help and advice for themselves, including consideration of the most constructive role for family members in self-exclusion and other forms of harm reduction

The need to change the ordinary business/responsible gambling ideology which has dominated official thinking about gambling regulation

I have argued that the *Gambling Establishment* has had a particular way of thinking about gambling which it has been endeavouring to implant in the public's mind. It is very easy to accept that way of thinking without reflection or resistance unless it is recognised for what it is – a set of assumptions which is very different from the one that prevailed only a very few decades ago. In Chapter 3, I tried to spell out what those assumptions are. The central one is that the business of providing gambling is an ordinary one, just like any other entertainment business. Another central *Gambling Establishment* assumption, which we were in the process of blindly accepting, is that gambling is inherently safe. The corollary of this is that any problems that do arise are confined to a very small minority who are not using the product responsibly. The consequences of accepting those assumptions uncritically are immense. They imply an open competitive market, advertising and welcoming technological innovation.

Sitting well with notions of gambling supply and consumption as ordinary business, harmless amusement and free choice is the powerful 'responsible gambling' philosophy with has dominated official thinking about gambling regulation since the run up to the 2005 Gambling Act. It is slowly becoming realised that this puts far too great an onus of responsibility for harm onto consumers and far too little on those who benefit financially from providing gambling and those responsible for allowing it. This has served the aims of promoting an expansionist gambling industry and distracting from criticism of its products.

The alternative: the dangerous consumption/public health perspective

The starting point for a new public discourse about gambling should be a recognition that gambling is not simply an ordinary entertainment product. Gambling, by its very nature, has always had the potential to be dangerously addictive. This has always been known. It is also tacitly acknowledged by gambling providers and the rest of the *Gambling Establishment* when they agree that, in order to be socially responsible, the offer of gambling should be accompanied by provision for harm reduction procedures such as self-exclusion and pre-commitment to spend or time limits. Modern forms of gambling are so dangerous that it is now judged to be irresponsible to provide them without at the same time having in place surveillance systems to detect harmful patterns of behaviour and schemes that help customers control their consumption. This is clearly no ordinary commodity we are talking about.

That acknowledgement of gambling's dangerousness should lead to the adoption of a public health perspective on gambling regulation. This would be new for Britain although the idea has been around for some time, particularly in countries such as Canada and New Zealand (e.g. Messerlian *et al.*, 2004). It should be adopted in the UK and be the basis for an international agreement. The UK, instead of being a world leader in providing online gambling, could become a world leader in terms of responsible government policy.

Globally, there is nothing about gambling to compare with WHO's (2010) *Global Strategy to Reduce the Harmful Use of Alcohol* or its stronger WHO (2003) *Framework Convention on Tobacco Control*. One set of international principles for gambling has been proposed by a group from Auckland, New Zealand (Adams, 2016). This *International Charter for Gambling* is based on the ideas of rights to freedom from harm and governments' duties of care and protection. Amongst other things, it states that regulation and policy should be set within 'a framework of independence from parties with a financial interest in the provision of gambling' and that gambling products and practices and their promotion should not be 'unduly exploitative or manipulative'. As we have seen, those are precisely the conditions that do not apply currently in Britain.

A similar suggestion, in the European Union context, was put forward by a group at the University of Helsinki. They have suggested pursuing harmonisation across Europe but within a framework of common EU values and goals, with an overriding aim of preventing harm and promoting social welfare and the common good by protecting the whole population. An important element would be separating financial interests from gambling policy and freeing regulation from the 'conflicts of interests as well as moral inconsistency' which has afflicted policy in Britain as well as in almost all other European systems of gambling regulation (Marionneau *et al.*, 2018).

There needs to be a national strategy for gambling with Government standing up to its responsibilities to protect its citizens from harm

A central problem has been Government's reluctance to get properly involved. Its policy has been to leave it to the industry to clean up its own act and pay for the damage caused. As the extent of the harm becomes clearer and the reluctance of the industry to making any significant changes that would impact on their profits becomes more evident, that strategy looks increasingly unfit for purpose. However, it is not clear that the present (as I write Conservative) UK Government wants to change it. The following revealing and worrying statement appeared in its 2017 consultation document (Department for Digital, Culture, Media and Sport, 2017b) which made it clear that it intends to continue to take a back seat, giving the industry a central position:

> we want to see industry, regulator and charities continue to drive the social responsibility agenda, to ensure that all is being done to protect players without the need for further Government intervention

On the contrary, I believe there is a need for a proper national Government strategy for gambling as there is for other types of dangerous consumption such as tobacco, alcohol and drugs. Bodies such as the Institute for Public Policy Research agree. In the IPPR (2016) report on the public costs of gambling-related harm, it also called for a national Government strategy to tackle problem gambling and reduce gambling-related harm. However, the necessary actions will not be taken if Government continues to take a back seat, leaving the protection of players and the public to industry, regulators and charities without the need for further Government intervention, as at present.

By a national gambling strategy, I mean one that comes from Government itself, not one emanating from an advisory body such as the Advisory Board for Safer Gambling (ABSG, until 2019 called the Responsible Gambling Strategy Board, RGSB) or the gambling regulator, the Gambling Commission (GC) in Britain's case. RGSB issued its own strategy document for 2016–19 which has sometimes been mistakenly construed as a national strategy. In 2019, the GC undertook to produce what it also called a national strategy. But ABSG/RGSB is, or at least should be, independent of Government, and the GC, as is appropriate for the regulator, likes to preserve its 'arm's length' separation from Government. The fact that both bodies have been so closely tied in with Government and industry as loyal constituents of the *Gambling Establishment*, and their confusion about where a national Government strategy should be coming from, are indications, if ever more were needed, that the system has been a broken one.

Until the surge in publicity around Government's reluctance to act on the FOBT machines (see Chapter 1), there had been no serious concerted political opposition in Britain to the continued growth of commercialised gambling, including the invention and forceful advertising of ever more addictive ways of gambling. Individual members of both Houses of Parliament had been sympathetic to groups such as the Campaign for Fairer Gambling, which had campaigned vigorously against the high-stake *fob-tees*, but neither of the two major political parties had deviated in any significant way from the Establishment line. Some Labour politicians who were around at that time have since admitted that the 2005 Act was a mistake, but official Labour Party policy had remained complicit with the well-entrenched Establishment view of things, until in 2017 the Labour Party brought out its radically different and more far-ranging proposals, including support for a new Gambling Act.

Gambling should be seen in Government as a cross-department issue with the health ministry playing a much larger, leading role

The 2016 IPPR report suggested that a national Government strategy should involve not only the Digital, Culture, Media and Sport department, as at present, but also other relevant Government departments. Problem gambling, they said, should be seen as a public health issue, and the Department of Health needed to start to take an interest in the subject, which they had failed to do to date. I agree. Gambling should be seen in Government as a cross–department issue, with at least the departments responsible for Health and Social Care, for Digital, Culture, Media and Sport, for Housing, Communities and Local Government, and for Education, plus the Home Office, each having regular and ongoing inputs.

Which of those government departments takes the lead on gambling in any country says a lot about the policy philosophy of that country's Establishment (see Chapter 2). One can think of two contrasting perspectives. The first sees gambling as an ordinary entertainment product linked to business, sport and culture. Since that was the dominant view, and Britain had a Department for Culture, Media and Sport (now Digital, Culture, Media and Sport), that department had a good claim to lead on the subject. The contrasting perspective sees gambling as a commodity dangerous to health. In Government, the Minister with chief responsibility for gambling should be a Department of Health Minister, reflecting an important shift towards seeing gambling first and foremost as a public health matter.

This is much more than just a dull point about government bureaucracy. It is crucial for understanding and correcting how the present unsatisfactory state of affairs has come about. Where gambling was placed in Government has been crucial for maintaining *Gambling Establishment* thinking. Yet when the British Government transferred responsibility to Culture, Media and Sport at the turn of the century, it was done quietly with no fanfare and scarcely any media attention. Power was being exercised, but the powerless were not informed.

Policy formation and the funding of gambling harm prevention, treatment and research must be completely independent of the industry

There is now widespread agreement about the need to avoid industry influence on the funding of gambling harm prevention, treatment and research (PT&R) and on policy formation generally. But so dominated has the *Gambling Establishment* been by industry interests, and so comparatively muted has been opposition to its thinking, that it lags far behind other similar fields in its consciousness about conflicts of interest (see Chapter 8). There is far greater recognition in relation to alcohol, for example, that policy formation as well as the funding of PT&R should be independent of the industry. As Margaret Chan, then Director General of the World Health Organisation, said in 2013 about the role of the alcohol industry in policy: 'In the view of WHO, the alcohol industry has no role in the formulation of alcohol policies, which must be protected from distortion by commercial or vested interests'.

The lack of proper independence is particularly serious when it comes to research. Because of the way in which gambling research is controlled by the industry in Britain, we are now losing out to other countries. There was a time when it looked as if Britain would be in the lead, at least as far as carrying out national population gambling surveys was concerned, having been one of the first countries to conduct two such studies. In fact, we were the first to have carried out three surveys, which provided a solid basis for beginning to look at trends over time. That lead was lost because Government withdrew funding for further dedicated gambling surveys, preferring the cheaper option of placing a much smaller number of questions about gambling in general health surveys.

Britain is now in danger of losing some of its best gambling research talent. Professor Luke Clark, who carried out some intriguing research on the subjective and brain effects of near-miss experiences on gambling machines when he was in Cambridge, was recruited as director of the new Centre for Gambling Research at the University of British Columbia in Canada. He has explained some of his thinking when deciding whether to accept that position (Clark, 2015), including obtaining assurance that he would have full independence in deciding on the new centre's research programme, and his lack of success when he was at Cambridge in obtaining an FOBT machine from the industry for research purposes.

This is the crucial issue of research access. It should not only include access to gambling venues and products but also access to 'internal industry working documents, such as industry-funded research reports and analysis' (Hancock, 2016). Research on tobacco offers a good example of how access to industry documents led to valuable studies exposing the exploitative and manipulative actions of companies: over 13 million industry documents were handed over which now form the Legacy Tobacco Documents Library, a valuable research resource (Adams, 2016). It may be unrealistic to expect something on that scale in the case of gambling in the near future, but the general point is a good one. The Establishment has no difficulty welcoming research that focuses on individual gamblers in trouble. If research which focuses on industry actors themselves as part of the problem is less welcome, what does that say about the influence the industry holds over the research agenda and its central position in the *Gambling Establishment*?

Funding gambling harm prevention, treatment and research: an industry levy?

Since the 2005 Gambling Act, Britain has suffered from a very unsatisfactory arrangement for funding gambling PT&R (incidentally, I put prevention first, although in practice it has been coming a poor third). Consistent with its taking-a-back-seat stance on gambling addiction and harm, Government decided to pass responsibility for this to the gambling industry. Gambling PT&R is funded from a voluntary levy on gambling companies. Contributions are purely voluntary, and the total amount raised annually – somewhat short of the £10 million target (The Telegraph, 2019) – is very far from adequate. Before considering what figure might be more appropriate, let us consider the question of whether a levy on the industry is the right way of raising the money. Opinions about this differ. Writing in an issue of an academic journal that looked specifically at research funding, one pair of commentators saw no good reason why funding should not come from the proceeds of gambling, 'as long as there is no prospect whatever of industry involvement, participation or public relations benefit' (Daube & Stoneham, 2016).

Other commentators drew a different conclusion. Some thought that, although independence from industry influence might be achieved despite gambling industry being the main source of funding, dependence on a flourishing industry for funding itself builds in a conflict of interest, and there remains an ethical issue since a very sizable proportion of income would thereby be coming from the pockets of people being harmed by gambling. Drawing on his own New Zealand experience, Peter Adams (2016, p 122) is also suspicious of claims or guarantees of no industry influence:

> On the surface, imposing hypothecated tax in the form of a levy on addictive consumptions, sometimes called 'earmarked taxes' or 'sin taxes', seems a very sensible way to address the wide range of associated health and social harms. . . [but] appearances can be deceptive. . . . The agency or department that manages hypothecated funding has the capacity to become a major, if not *the* major, voice on issues relating to these products. . . [because it] . . . is positioned within or alongside the government sector and. . . [has] access to levy funds to resource their own operations.

My own conclusion continues to be that funding gambling PT&R out of general taxation would be the right way: that would clearly establish the field as an essential one equivalent to others of public health importance, independent of the industry. If there were to continue to be a levy, it should be mandatory, not voluntary, and should be set much higher than the present target in order to more adequately cover the needs and to bring spending more in line with other countries.

What would be a more reasonable figure? An alternative basis for arriving at a target could be an estimate of the proportion of Gross Gambling Yield (GGY) which is contributed by people with gambling disorder. Survey findings suggest the adult 12-month prevalence of gambling disorder is about 7–8 per 1,000, or just under 1%, with at least twice that number at significant risk due to the way they are gambling (Gambling Commission, 2019b; Wardle *et al.*, 2011). Because they spend more than the average, the percentage of GGY which they contribute is much higher than the prevalence estimate, although secondary analysis of the 2010 British Gambling Prevalence Survey data suggested it varies greatly by type of gambling (from around 5% for bingo and football pools gambling to around 25% for betting on dog races and playing FOBTs) (Orford *et al.*, 2013). In total, the estimate was that around 10% of takings on all forms of gambling regulated by the Gambling Commission come from people with gambling problems (we were deliberately cautious in arriving at these estimates; others, such as the Australian Productivity Commission, 1999, have put the figure much higher).

Given our conservative estimates that nearly 1% of adults have gambling disorder and that they contribute at least 10% of GGY, £10 million (about 0.1% of GGY) as a levy target looks paltry. Bearing in mind that only a proportion of GGY translates into industry profits, 1% of current GGY, or around £140 million, might be a more reasonable figure. This puts the present target of £10 million into proper perspective. Not only is it a pitifully small amount in relation to PT&R needs, but it is also nowhere near what is reasonable in relation to the prevalence of problem gambling and the percentage of industry profits coming from people with gambling problems.

In short, the present British system of financing gambling PT&R through a small annual voluntary levy administered by a body, GambleAware, close to the gambling industry and with industry origins, does not command respect and should be reformed. Government should face up to its responsibility to adequately fund gambling PT&R from general taxation. In the light of Sulkunen *et al.*'s (2019) calculation that gambling in the UK contributes a relatively small amount to the Government treasury compared to other countries (see Chapter 2), it would be reasonable to consider raising gambling taxes. Alternatively there should be a mandatory levy, including a proportionate contribution from National Lottery takings, substantially increased in size and administered by a body that is completely independent of the industry – a principle which is established without question in other public health fields.

By whatever means the funds are raised, through direct taxation – my preference – or via a mandatory levy, the most important thing is that decisions about allocating these resources should be made by an independent body set up for the purpose: possibly a National Institute or a Gambling Council to which organisations conducting PT&R would be able to bid openly for funding. It would be similar in some ways to the Research Councils. The present situation regarding the funding of research is particularly unsatisfactory and must be changed if the field is to gain credibility, if sound research is to be carried out and young talent is to be attracted to the area.

The issue of advertising, and especially television advertising and sports sponsorship, should be reconsidered

As we saw in Chapter 4, the quantity and content of gambling advertising are particularly contentious issues, especially in a country like Britain that has a regime that is one of the most accommodating of gambling advertising. Advertising is the facet of modern gambling's normalisation which is most apparent to members of the general public. The television advertising of gambling is not the only aspect, but it is one that is arousing special concern. The protection of children and young people is one of the three main principles underlying the regulatory work of the Gambling Commission. The showing on television prior to the 9.00 pm 'watershed' of encouragements to gamble, both on the outcome of the sporting event being shown and on in-play bets, at a time when children and young people are very likely to be excited about watching a sporting event in the company of family members, is arguably putting children and young people at risk in a way that should concern the Gambling Commission. The anomaly of pre-watershed advertising of gambling allowed in Britain is another good example of a policy strongly lobbied for by gambling providers that was allowed to slip in without national debate. In the previous chapter we saw how, since then, evidence has been used in a highly selective way to support the perpetuation of that unpopular policy. The precautionary principle should prevail here. Prevention of harm should take precedence over other considerations.

The complete removal of gambling advertising on TV before the evening watershed would be a very popular move. The industry is aware of this and has taken some small steps in the right direction. In 2014, the Senet group, an industry group set up to promote responsible gambling, voluntarily agreed not to advertise the offer of free bets before 9.00 pm (The Drum, 2014). Then, towards the end of 2018, with gambling advertising associated with televised football matches under increasing criticism, some of the biggest UK betting companies announced their intention to institute a 'whistle to whistle' ban on adverts during sporting events such as football matches starting before 9.00 pm. This was welcomed by some, but in reality what they proposed didn't go anywhere near far enough, amounting to simply removing adverts during the halftime break. In the total picture of how much coverage these huge companies get, the so-called 'whistle to whistle' ban on adverts is trivial. Much more useful to the companies are the sponsorship deals with the big football clubs, the adverts carried on moving banners around the grounds and on players' shirts, and logos appearing behind players and managers when interviewed at the grounds on highlights shows like the BBC's *Match of the Day*, not to mention all their public, online and social media–linked advertising.

Similar moves imposed by governments had been announced earlier in some other countries, including Australia and Belgium. The Australian move included banning adverts from five minutes before to five minutes after a match, which is an improvement. But that was also criticised as not being sufficient to address the problem. The Belgium proposal would ban any gambling advertising during live sports broadcasts and within 15 minutes before or after any programmes aimed at minors, use in adverts of athletes or celebrities with particular appeal for minors, and advertisements via platforms or media targeted mainly at minors. In February 2019, the Committees of Advertising Practice (CsAP) in Britain also proposed enforcing similar rules about separating gambling advertising from programmes, celebrities or media aimed at children (iGaming Business, 2019b). But this amounts to a necessary enforcement of existing regulations, not the kind of real change that is necessary.

The minimum change that is needed to protect children and young people is a ban on any gambling promotion which is especially likely to be seen or heard by under-18s. This would require not only a proper pre-watershed ban on television advertising to include the crucial pre-match period but also removal of all gambling advertising visible during sporting fixtures popular with children and young people. That would in effect mean outlawing gambling company sponsorship of football and other sporting teams as has happened in a number of other countries such as Germany, Portugal, France and the Netherlands (Banks, 2014).

This would be resisted by some. But it would be popular with many, including many parents and carers. It would also be consistent with the positive health and well-being enhancing community work which many clubs engage in. The wholesale encouragement of sports gambling, which has become the norm and which clubs have been contributing to, is encouraging the development of habits which are putting young people at risk of current and future harm, working in a direction counter to clubs' valuable community work. Removing gambling advertising and sponsorship which impacts children and young people would also send a strong message to them and those who care for them, and to everyone else, that gambling is a public health issue and that Government takes seriously its responsibility to protect the young and to promote cultural practices consistent with the general good.

The protection of children and young people should be the first consideration when the issue of advertising is reconsidered in the course of drawing up proposals for a new Gambling Act and formulating a new national gambling strategy. When that is done, advertising should be dealt with thoroughly in all its forms. In Chapter 4, I highlighted not only the danger of gambling becoming increasingly aligned with sport but also the 'aggressive' promotion of online gambling and the new grey area of gambling and gambling-like games and links on social media. The introduction of children to gambling through social media should be examined especially closely and appropriate measures taken.

In the UK, the Advertising Standards Authority (ASA) oversees and implements the CsAP codes governing gambling advertising. Among its list of rules are some obvious ones such as rules against encouraging criminality or appealing to sexual success or toughness and others that are more subtle and open to interpretation. The latter include the strictures that advertising must not portray, condone or encourage gambling that could lead to financial, social or emotional harm; suggest that gambling can be a solution to financial concerns; be likely to be of particular appeal to children or young persons, especially by reflecting or being associated with youth culture; or exploit cultural beliefs or traditions about gambling or luck. The public is exhorted to report individual adverts which it is thought might be in breach of any of the rules. That misses the point. The way gambling has come to be advertised in the modern era breaks those rules constantly. It is the rules themselves that need to be reconsidered from scratch in the light of the radically new way of viewing the place of gambling in society which a new Gambling Act and national gambling strategy would usher in.

Swedish social scientist Per Binde (2009), the acknowledged expert on gambling advertising whom we met in earlier chapters, has made his own recommendations about responsible gambling advertising. In his opinion it should not target vulnerable groups such as the poor, young people and problem gamblers; should not suggest that it is a way to solve economic problems nor encourage excessive gambling; should not claim that gambling is risk-free; and should not be aggressive by occupying excessive media space or adopting a hard-sell tone. The subjectively misleading aspect of gambling advertising could be countered, he suggested, by companies providing easily accessible information on how games work. It should be more transparent about the chances of winning and the net cost of gambling, and this information should be displayed in advertising and at points of sale and printed on lottery and betting tickets. His recommendations would provide a good starting point for a complete rethink about the way in which gambling might be advertised more responsibly in Britain and elsewhere. It is unlikely that reverting to a time when all gambling advertising was banned, as the Italian Government has decreed (Daily Mail, 2018b), would be supported, but, as politicians are fond of saying, all options should be on the table.

Harm reduction

HR: Why the gambling-providing industry is ambivalent about it

Most of my other suggestions can be subsumed under the general heading of *harm reduction*, or HR. The core idea, the master narrative if you will, behind the power of the *Gambling Establishment* has been that of 'responsible gambling', as discussed in Chapter 3. This has profound implications when it comes to harm reduction. For a start, the industry seems to prefer the term 'harm minimisation'. That might suggest that harm is a relatively minor issue which can be kept to a minimum or that policy should aim to accommodate or adjust to dangers rather than adopt a critical stance towards the existing arrangements which give rise to dangers (Cantinotti & Ladouceur, 2008). The former is likely to emphasise strengthening individuals in coping with the dangers. The latter is more likely to support social and political action to influence governments and commercial decision-making. Needless to say, the former is more attractive to the Establishment which supports the status quo.

Those who have thought hard about HR theory have pointed out that it can be narrowly or broadly defined (Weatherburn, 2009). The narrow definition restricts it to measures that do not in themselves affect the supply or demand of the consumption product. For example, serving beer in plastic rather than glass containers in an effort to minimise serious injuries resulting from alcohol-related fights is unlikely to have much effect on alcohol consumption. Likewise, providing counselling for large National Lottery winners is not likely to affect NL takings. There are probably very few measures which fit the narrow definition of HR. Most measures designed to reduce problem gambling are also likely to reduce overall gambling through their effect on demand or supply. They are therefore resisted by the providing industry. Hence the resistance of the alcohol industry to unit pricing, the resistance of the Australian machine gambling industry to mandatory pre-commitment (see later in this chapter) and the resistance of the British betting industry to the reduction in maximum stake size on fixed odds betting machines. There is a fundamental contradiction in the idea of the gambling-providing industry embracing HR. Along with governments and the rest of the *Gambling Establishment*, they believe they can promote a liberalised industry and at the same time seriously undertake HR. They want to have their cake and eat it. This is a fiction. The Establishment is bound to be ambivalent about HR. So long as measures offer no serious threat to industry takings, they will be at least considered. If they are a threat to profits – and all but a very narrow band of measures do offer some threat – they will be resisted.

The Gambling Establishment favours gambling education, the weakest form of prevention

Of the many gambling HR methods that are possible and which are in operation in one jurisdiction or another, some may give the impression that they are effective while at the same time being neutral in terms of industry takings and contribution to government finances. At the least Establishment-challenging end of the political-versus-personal, critical-versus-accommodationist spectrum are educational approaches, including some that are school-based and others aimed at the population in general. This is classic primary prevention, and it sounds as if it makes good sense. It is often the first thing people think of when asked for their opinions about how something like problem gambling can be prevented. And it is certainly what the *Gambling Establishment* wants to emphasise. In fact it has often used the word 'education' as a synonym for 'prevention' as if educating young people and adults about responsible gambling was the only sensible way in which harm could be prevented. It has the appearance of being positive and humane. It is relatively uncontroversial. And most important of all, it leaves intact and unaddressed the development and promotion of the commodities that are causing the problems in the first place.

Unfortunately, education is one of the weakest forms of prevention, and it doesn't work well. The results are very much the same as those found in the case of alcohol and drugs – it can have an immediate effect on knowledge and attitudes, but its longer term effects on behaviour are minimal (Orford, 2013). In the case of gambling, it can be successful in reducing misconceptions about gambling, increasing knowledge of problem gambling, and changing attitudes towards gambling, but it meets with limited success in reducing subsequent gambling behaviour (Ariyabuddhiphongs, 2013). It is ideally suited to giving the impression that something is being done without threatening profits. At best it is naive. Worse, it may be cynical – engaging in ineffectual conversations with people about a dangerous activity while continuing to make money out of people's addiction to it.

Worst of all, gambling education may well be counterproductive. The encouragement to gamble sensibly or responsibly actually contains two messages: one, the apparent surface message, encouraging behaving sensibly or responsibly; the other, the latent message, that to gamble is acceptable and normal. Educational approaches, particularly in a developing or expanding market, may actually be making matters worse, not better.

Tracking and identifying problem players: an ill-conceived and ineffective form of HR

One approach to HR which is favoured by the *Gambling Establishment* is that of identifying problem players. This has several advantages for the industry. It puts the spotlight directly on individual players rather than on what the providers are providing for them to gamble on. It is one of the most individualistic and, from the industry perspective, least threatening of all HR approaches. It fits with that part of the Establishment discourse which claims that only a small minority of people are unable or unwilling to manage their gambling without harm. And if in the process it can identify some of its more troublesome customers – for example those who make a nuisance of themselves by kicking out at gambling machines or sending angry messages to online gambling companies – so much the better.

The more positive spin on this is to say that the industry and its venue staff have an obligation to try and identify and assist customers who may be getting into trouble with their gambling. But would venue staff know enough about individual customers to know whether they need help or not? A Swiss study (Häfeli & Schneider, 2006) which involved interviews with both casino employees and gambling patrons produced a list of no less than 39 possible indicators of problems such as excessive time and money spent gambling, raising additional funds by using ATMs or borrowing, making large or high-risk bets, negative social behaviour such as rudeness or avoidance of social contact, and a general behaviour category which included such things as strong emotional responses to losing, the use of superstitious rituals, and signs of stress and anxiety such as shaking and excessive sweating. A number of casinos, such as Sky City Auckland in New Zealand, have developed similar lists of indicators (Ward, 2012).

Some of the best studies of how identification works in practice have been Australian. One particularly thorough multi-method series of studies (Delfabbro *et al.*,

2011) confirmed that many of these indicators were significantly more likely to be reported by players who had problems with their gambling. But an observational study suggested that there were several impediments to successful identification. For example, staff often spent a quarter or less of their time on the gaming floor, and it was only possible to accumulate enough evidence by watching individual gamblers for many hours at a time or over multiple sessions. Another of these studies pointed to a number of realities regarding what goes on in EGM venues and the position that venue staff are placed in with regard to the personal harm being done to many of their customers. Of those who were familiar to venue staff as regulars, 15% were thought to have at least some problems with their gambling. But in the large majority of such cases, although staff believed there probably was a problem, they could not be confident about it. As the authors of the report said, 'there are likely to be significant challenges associated with using observational methods to identify problem gamblers within venues.'

In the case of online gambling, it is easier to monitor actual gambling behaviour such as the frequency and size of bets and escalation in staking. This offers the apparently perfect opportunity to 'track' gamblers' behaviour, potentially collect and analyse colossal amounts of data – apparent heaven to psychologists like me – and identify abnormal patterns of play. However, the faith that the Establishment has been placing in online gambling 'player tracking' is misplaced. Preliminary evidence of that was discussed in the previous chapter, and further such evidence comes from the second phase of the GambleAware commissioned machines research. The report said they had, 'found the industry could accurately detect problem gamblers. . . [providing] a key area of opportunity for operators to strengthen their processes to identify and minimise gambling-related harm' (GambleAware, 2017a). Unfortunately, that statement is greatly over-optimistic. Close reading of the report of that work, available on the GambleAware website, in fact shows that, even when 22 indicators are put into the equation, the degree to which users of online gambling sites who are otherwise thought to have gambling problems (because of their answers to the Problem Gambling Severity Index) could be identified was very far from perfect. The overall most accurate prediction still produced an unacceptably high proportion of false positives and false negatives. There is the further problem that complicated algorithms of this sort are likely to become even less accurate over time as gambling products, environments and players change.

One of the other things about player tracking and identification of problem players generally is what the implications might be for privacy and surveillance. On several occasions I have raised with representatives of the Gambling Commission the question of whether all this has implications for safeguarding consumer privacy. Is this even a human rights issue, I wonder? My questions about this are usually met with surprise and incomprehension. Meanwhile, the Commission was looking forward to the time when identification of problem players in the case of non-remote or 'land-based' gambling would be made much easier with the help of facial-recognition technology! It seems never to have occurred to the *Gambling*

Establishment that its attempts to 'minimise' harm from gambling are in themselves proof of how dangerous these 'products' are and, in the process, may also be contributing to reinforcing our surveillance society.

The establishment bias in HR is towards individual self-control: self-exclusion, time-outs and voluntary loss limit setting as examples

In Britain the Gambling Commission has included self-exclusion as a licencing requirement since 2007. Self-excluders and potential self-excluders are often critical of the lax way in which self-exclusion has operated in practice. Recommendations for improvement include the need for operators to have an effective training programme for all staff and to suspend marketing and incentives for all self-excluded people, both requirements which have often not been met in practice. Most important is the need to be able to exclude oneself from multiple venues, not just a single venue (Gainsbury, 2014). The Commission promised to have such a one-stop shop in force by the end of 2015, at least in each of the gambling industry sectors separately, with ambitions for a cross-sector scheme shortly thereafter. GamStop, the industry-run scheme that resulted from that initiative, took longer to get off the ground than was hoped, starting in April 2018 and reported in a BBC investigation to be still having teething troubles in January 2019 (iGaming Business, 2019a). Meanwhile, Gamban had started up as a non-industry alternative.

In fact, the Gambling Commission (2015) has described self-exclusion as just one of a number of 'gambling management tools' – an interesting expression which fits well with the assumption that, should problems arise with your use of commercial gambling products, it is your own faulty management which is to blame, and we can help you manage it better (see Chapter 3). The Commission considered it more efficient to have other mechanisms in place 'to deal with problems before they arise and to offer players tools to help manage their gambling responsibly'. One of these is 'time-outs', which were supported by the industry-led Responsible Gambling Trust as an alternative to self-exclusion, giving players more choice. In a way this would be rather like a short self-exclusion – 24 hours, one week, one month – for those at risk of developing 'harmful gambling habits'. Significantly, the suggestion was that this would not involve cessation of marketing.

It is not difficult to appreciate why the industry would be more in favour of brief time-outs as opposed to full self-exclusions. Only the latter recognises the serious difficulties that some people are in with regard to their gambling and the need for a thoroughgoing break from gambling. From an industry perspective, brief time-outs, which give the appearance of recognising a person's gambling problem, serve to maintain the relationship between gambling providers and some of their most profitable customers with just a short break and no curtailment of marketing. This is a good example of a policy that is dressed up as serious HR but which in reality is likely to be an ineffective policy mainly serving the interests of the industry. It underlines the point that an industry which has been allowed to operate in the free market is bound to favour weak rather than strong forms of HR.

The other Establishment-favoured self-control HR method is making provision for customers to set their own gambling limits, usually a limit on the amount that can be lost in a session of gambling and/or sometimes a time limit. This is usually referred to as 'pre-commitment'. The operator is required to respect the stated limit and to withhold the opportunity to gamble further once the limit is reached. This is intriguing, and goes to the heart of thorny questions about the nature of gambling and how to reduce its harms. Commercial gambling requires most customers to lose; otherwise winnings could not be paid out and profits could not be made. Understandably, gambling companies are ambivalent about loss limits, which is why the Australian industry devoted so much of its resources to opposing the stronger form of limit setting – *mandatory* limits. That would have required operators to insist that all players set limits before they could begin to gamble. The industry won, and Australia now has the weaker voluntary system that simply requires operators to ask if a player wishes to set a limit – apparently few accept the invitation.

Mandatory pre-commitment, stronger though it is, still qualifies as a self-control form of HR; the onus is still on the individual gambler to set the limit or limits. There is a yet stronger form of limit setting, operating, for example, in the Netherlands, in parts of Germany and in part of the gambling sector in Finland. This does not invite or require customers to set their own limits but imposes absolute limits on all customers, for example restricting total amounts of losses or maximum total online bets per hour, day, week or month. This in effect promotes limit setting from a self-control HR method to one which modifies the product. It does that in a way which, it can be argued, is consistent with the Establishment claim that gambling is a form of entertainment. If that is the case, then it is not unreasonable that there should be a maximum price for the entertainment. This is the strongest form of limit setting, the most challenging to industry interests and therefore likely to be hotly resisted. Some combination of absolute and mandatory-self-chosen limit setting should be included as part of a new Gambling Strategy for Britain.

Whether in the form of self-exclusion, time-outs or setting loss limits, the underlying philosophy, consistent with the Reno Model and *Gambling Establishment* thinking generally, has been that the way to carry on promoting gambling whilst 'minimising' its harmful consequences is to help individual gamblers control themselves. The aim is to try and identify individuals with problems, to give them self-control tools and, if really necessary, exclude them, preferably voluntarily. This has the obvious industry advantage of distracting attention from the inherent dangers of the product and the ways it is promoted.

Stronger forms of HR which challenge the Gambling Establishment

When it comes to HR methods which are potentially stronger and less accommodating of gambling-provider interests, there is no shortage of ideas. I often meet the suggestion that little can be done to stem the continued expansion of gambling, especially online gambling. In fact there are numerous things that can be done and indeed are being done somewhere in the world (Ariyabuddhiphongs, 2013; Dickerson & O'Connor, 2006; Dickson–Gillespie *et al.*, 2008; Wood *et al.*, 2014). There is no excuse for inaction.

Two comprehensive reviews of the effectiveness of HR strategies have been carried out, the first in 2007 (Williams *et al.*, 2007) and the second 10 years later (Tanner *et al.*, 2017); and one of the most thorough summaries of the global evidence on gambling HR is contained in the publication *Setting Limits: Gambling, Science, and Public Policy* (Sulkunen *et al.*, 2019). Evaluation research concerning most HR methods has either not yet been carried out or has produced mixed or unclear results. Hence the reviews are rarely able to come up with unequivocal recommendations. Even the popular self-exclusion has met with mixed reviews, although the conclusion of one particularly thorough review was that the majority of participants do benefit (Gainsbury, 2014). There are some obvious problems with HR evaluation. One is that preventing gambling harm, and researching the effectiveness of trying to do so, has simply not been a sufficiently high enough priority. Good research is expensive, and that is particularly the case when trying to evaluate preventive efforts since it generally requires following people up for long enough to be able to tell whether prevention has worked. Extra complication is added due to the fact that so much of the detail about forms of gambling, laws and regulations, not to mention local social and cultural practices and attitudes, vary so much from place to place. Innovation, technology and policy are also fast moving. This all makes it difficult to pinpoint the exact causes of any changes observed or be sure whether results obtained in one country at one time would apply elsewhere or at a later time.

The 2019 *Setting Limits* review was able to reach a number of general conclusions, however. The first was that HR measures which modify features of gambling product design are more effective than those that aim to identify and influence individual players. This supports the general conclusion of those who have considered reducing the harms associated with other dangerous forms of consumption (Adams, 2016; Orford, 2013) and the conclusion I and others have reached about gambling HR specifically.

A second conclusion was that any changes made need to be of sufficient magnitude to be able to produce demonstrable effects. For example, on the specific issue of reducing maximum stake sizes for EGMs, based particularly on a comparison between relatively small reductions made in Victoria and South Australia and larger reductions made in Norway, the review concluded that to be effective in reducing harm the reductions had to be substantial.

A further conclusion from all the research they looked at is that several measures in combination are more effective than a single measure alone. Hence, reducing stake size is likely to be even more effective if combined with other measures taken simultaneously, such as increasing the minimum interval between plays, banning autoplay, reducing arousing visual and auditory stimulation, and setting mandatory loss limits. Nova Scotia is an example of a jurisdiction where a substantial proportion of EGMs, about 30%, were removed, combined with reduction in their service hours, leading to an overall decrease in machine playtime and a substantial reduction in expenditure (Corporate Research Associates, 2006). In the UK, the All Party Parliamentary Group (APPG) on the FOBTs also recommended that Government should consider, in addition to reducing maximum stake size, reducing the speed of operation of the machines, reviewing the use of debit cards and the use of the 'repeat' function, looking at the question of opening hours, reviewing levels of staffing, and devolving powers to local authorities to reduce clustering of bookmakers' shops.

Among other HR methods which have some support from international research are those that limit the ease with which those gambling can make large payments or top up their funds. This includes removing note acceptors, limiting access to credit, showing credits and losses in real money, paying winnings by cheque or vouchers instead of cash, removing ATMs from the immediate vicinity, and blocking bank account payments to gambling companies. Others involve removal of design features which encourage faulty cognitions and increase game intensity, such as restricting jackpot size or availability, sound and visual effects, near misses and LDWs (losses disguised as wins – see Chapter 5). Prohibiting or discouraging smoking and alcohol use in gambling venues is another.

Age restrictions

One of the clearest recommendations of one review was about legal age limits, which it concluded were generally effective (Gainsbury et al., 2014). Indeed, referring to work on executive brain functioning, which may still be developing throughout young adulthood (see Chapter 6), the review stated its opinion that a legal age of 18 years might be too low to protect adolescents and young adults and that it might be sensible to increase the legal age for gambling further, as in the USA, Greece, Belgium, Portugal and Singapore, perhaps to age 21. It is unlikely there would be public support in the UK for an increase to age 21, but there would probably be more support for implementing 18 as the legal age for gambling more consistently. There are at least two anomalies. The Gambling Review Body of 2001 thought allowing British children to play low-stake/low-prize EGMs was inconsistent with the principles that should govern modern gambling regulation, but in that case the 'seaside tradition' argument was successfully used to defend the status quo. Also under discussion has been the current exception of the National Lottery for which 16-year-olds can purchase tickets. Consideration should be given to having a minimum age of 18 years for all gambling, consistent with the general message that gambling is dangerous for children and young people. At the same time, age verification should be strengthened.

Two important principles: proper impact assessment and reduction in ambient gambling

There should be a full impact assessment of any proposed new form of gambling or change to an existing form of gambling

Any proposed new form of gambling, mode or type of venue should be subject to a full social, health and economic impact assessment. This would be designed to avoid the kind of mistake that was made when the new Fixed Odds Betting Terminals (FOBTs) form of EGMs were permitted in British betting shops. The lack of openness and transparency in the process of their introduction, the way in which promoters used their power and influence to head off tighter regulation, and the industry's control of subsequent research (see Chapter 8) are stark illustrations of how a large and powerful industry can get its way. It can and almost certainly will happen again unless new rules prevent it. The gambling-promoting industry has technology on its side. Its greatest asset is the collusion of the rest of the *Gambling Establishment*.

The FOBT saga also offers a perfect example of something that we have seen repeatedly in gambling policy. This is the process whereby an innovative form or mode of gambling, or relaxation of a previous regulation, is allowed in without a proper assessment of its likely impact, including impact on children and young people and other vulnerable sections of the population, and with little or no public debate. Thereafter, strong arguments are mounted against reversing the process. In the case of the FOBTs the argument for resisting greater control has rested in large part on the damage such control might do to employment in the betting industry – although the industry is already planning ways it can mitigate the change now that it is unavoidable (see Chapter 2).

No evidence about safety or consumer protection was required when FOBTs were introduced. The onus of proof is unfairly placed on those who speak for people who are harmed; it should be on those who profit from products of questionable safety and those who support their position. The ruling principle has been that because the provision of gambling is to be seen as an ordinary business like any other, innovation is to be welcomed and encouraged and only restricted when sufficient evidence has accumulated to be utterly convincing that safety is being compromised. What should have ruled instead is the precautionary principle – not to expose people to something that is potentially dangerous until it is proved to be safe.

Another false claim that has been used in defence of FOBTs is that no one form of gambling is any more harmful than any other. In Britain we have nothing for gambling similar to the Class A, B, C system which is central to regulation of illicit drug supply and consumption. In fact such systems do exist for suggesting how dangerous a form of gambling might be – the Veikkaus Ray model from Finland being one and social responsibility tools, such as AsTERiG and GamGard being others (Häfeli, 2014). Greater use should be made of these as a guide, and providers should be mandated to prove a product or venue is safe before it is launched.

Ambient gambling and local option

Two among the long list of existing HR methods are of special interest to those of us in the UK because they were both recommendations made by the Gambling Review Body (2001), which preceded the 2005 Gambling Act, but which were rejected by Government. Although the Review report was largely a very liberalising, industry-friendly one, one of its most basic principles was that what they called 'ambient gambling' should not be encouraged; in other words, that, by and large, gambling should be restricted to premises where gambling was the main activity. A good example was jackpot machines in private clubs, which the committee recommended should no longer be allowed. Government disagreed. Several years later, when the Department for Culture, Media and Sport Select Committee (House of Commons, 2012) reviewed how the 2005 Act had being working out – another largely complacent document – it pointed out that placing non-slots, casino-like, high-intensity FOBT EGMs outside casinos in highstreet betting shops was contrary to the 'regulatory pyramid' which Government has subscribed to in the past, under which the most intensive and dangerous forms of gambling were confined to the less accessible locations. This question of where different forms of 'land-based' gambling should be provided is of great salience in other countries, including in European countries such as Italy and in New Zealand and Australia, where it has been the proliferation of EGMs in bars, pubs and clubs that has been so controversial.

A related principle underlying the review committee's recommendations which was rejected was the idea of allowing local authorities greater say in what gambling would be provided in their areas. In fact, the Review Body had suggested that local authorities might have the power to ban particular types of gambling premises in particular areas or even to impose a ban on all gambling premises. This interesting idea of local option was rejected by Government and the idea has not resurfaced since. Local authorities are left with the very considerable and highly frustrating task of licencing gambling premises but with little real power to control what gambling is offered in their communities. Along with a clearer adherence to the principle of preventing ambient gambling, local option should be reconsidered.

There needs to be a proper comprehensive system of treatment for people with gambling problems and help for their families

Although gambling disorder is recognised as an ill-health condition by the World Health Organisation and other international bodies, treatment provision in Britain is currently sparse and inadequate. The Responsible Gambling Strategy Board

(2016), in their Strategy 2016–17 to 2018–19 document, said, 'the absence of any significant NHS treatment is striking'. This despite the figures suggesting that gambling problem prevalence is of the same order as the prevalence of problems related to the misuse of illicit drugs (European Monitoring Centre for Drugs and Drug Addiction, 2018). The latter, unlike gambling disorder, is recognised as a major public health problem for which health authorities have a responsibility to provide treatment. This is an issue in most other high income, well-resourced countries, the USA for one (Weinstock *et al.*, 2018). In less resourced countries the situation is even worse. The 'treatment gap' – the difference between the estimated prevalence of a health problem and the numbers receiving treatment for it – is particularly large in the case of gambling: as high as 95% in Britain according to figures produced by GambleAware (2017b).

Compared to work in other fields, such as the treatment of alcohol problems, the development and evaluation of gambling treatment is at an early stage. The best reviews include a Cochrane-style review which supported the efficacy of psychological therapy, specifically cognitive behaviour therapy (CBT) and motivational interviewing (MI), although there have as yet been few follow-up studies (Cowlishaw *et al.*, 2012). The longer established mutual help organisation Gamblers Anonymous (GA) also has an important role to play (Petry, 2005). Medications effective in the treatment of substance addictions and psychiatric disorders that can co-occur with problem gambling have also been used (Bullock & Potenza, 2015). Increasing the volume and quality of treatment research will be important.

As relevant as questions about the type of treatment are those to do with access to help, such as where treatment services for gambling problems are best located. One suggestion is that existing addiction/substance misuse services would be the best location. However, despite their expertise in treating addictive disorders, knowledge of gambling disorder and confidence in dealing with it is often surprisingly low within such services, and the treatment of gambling disorder, if provided for at all, is a low priority. The same is even more true in mental health services where gambling problems quite often present themselves. There remains a lot of work to do in raising consciousness about gambling problems among health and social service staff.

Since for many people with gambling disorder their problems are complex and associated with other mental and physical health difficulties, with domestic abuse and other family problems, with debt or with problems of social disadvantage, treatment for gambling problems must be well integrated with services that deal with those health and social problems. An important component of treatment for gambling problems is provision of financial counselling for people with debt or money-management problems related to gambling. A further important element is the recognition of gambling issues in the law enforcement, crime prevention and legal counselling systems and in homelessness services, as the clients of those services are known to have particularly high rates of gambling problems. Finally, such recognition should also be incorporated into services for children and young persons, including further and higher education students, as the prevalence of gambling problems is known to be as high if not higher among adolescents and young people than among adults (National Research Council, 1999).

An effective treatment system is likely to embrace a variety of approaches, ranging from hospital or community residential facilities, at the more intensive end of the spectrum, to brief, early interventions, telephone helplines and online support at the other extreme. Gambling helplines and e-help for gambling have been trialled in a number of countries, including Britain (Goh, 2017). Ideally, there should be a variety of ways in which people can obtain appropriate help, advice or an opportunity to discuss their concerns about their own gambling or about someone else's gambling. Early and preventive interventions targeted at risky gambling will be as important as treatments clearly designated for problem gambling.

Wherever treatment and support for gambling problems is located, it is unlikely to flourish without the stimulus and backup of at least a small number of specialist centres dedicated to the treatment of gambling problems. One such centre, operating under the umbrella of the NHS but, at least until recently, funded from the gambling industry levy, has been doing excellent work in London for a number of years. A second specialist NHS clinic, to serve Northern England, has been agreed and should be opening in 2019, and at least another two or three elsewhere in Britain would be useful. The specialist regional clinics should be centres for research and evaluation and training as much as for the routine provision of treatment. They would play an important role in raising awareness of gambling disorder and the profile of gambling problem treatment nationwide.

Affected family members should play a role in treatment and need help and advice for themselves

In Chapter 7, close family members of people with gambling problems were identified as one of the largest groups of people harmed by gambling. The stress associated with having a close relative adversely affected by gambling varies and can often be extreme, leading to mental health consequences for a family member: many would benefit from help for themselves in their own right. Many, perhaps the large majority, are affected by the gambling problem of a relative who is not currently receiving any formal treatment or help: they may need advice about how to cope and how to encourage their relatives to engage with assistance. When relatives are receiving treatment, family members have potential as important partners in their relatives' treatment and recovery.

It is now much better accepted than it was that services for people with psychological problems, not only addiction problems, should, as a matter of course, make effort to engage with family members. This has been recognised, for example, in the widespread adoption by British NHS mental health service providers of what is known as the Triangle Approach (Carers Trust, 2013). This is an acknowledgement of the evidence that there are three partners in the treatment of a psychological problem – the patient, the professional, and the family – and that it is in everyone's interest for them to work together.

In the case of addiction treatment, there is abundant evidence both that the patient's treatment is enhanced by family involvement (Ingle *et al.*, 2008; Jiménez-Murcia *et al.*, 2016) and that affected family members benefit from help in their own right. Among methods for engaging and helping affected family members, the most generally applicable is the 5-Step Method, developed in the UK and used at the National Problem Gambling Clinic in London, in Australia, and with those affected by addiction problems generally in a number of other countries, Ireland being one (Copello *et al.*, 2010; Orford *et al.*, 2017).

Family members' role in exclusion

One further specific issue is the role of affected family members in exclusion. More careful thought needs to be given to this. It is not sufficient, and is certainly not consistent with the Triangle Approach philosophy, to say that exclusion has nothing to do with affected family members. There are several steps that may be of help to a worried member of the family impotently witnessing what is happening to a loved one and/or to family life. The first is information. Affected family members may know little about self-exclusion, and the more they know the more help they can be to their relatives. A second step is advice about how best to encourage a relative to consider and embark on self-exclusion. A third is consideration of more active steps to promote exclusion, as happens in a number of countries such as Germany and Singapore (Goh *et al.*, 2016; Kotter *et al.*, 2018), for example by approaching the staff and management of a gambling venue to discuss how best to help one of their customers who may already be of concern to venue staff. Part of a national strategy for gambling should be consideration of the best constructive role for family members in harm reduction, including in self-exclusion. This is not happening in Britain at the moment.

Conclusion

This brings me to the end of my recommendations for change and to the conclusion of the book as a whole. Gambling has been allowed to encroach more and more on our lives. I hope I have been able to show how aware we need to be about how this has happened. My thesis has been that we were steadily being conditioned to accept gambling's enlarged place in society, and that this conditioning – brainwashing if you will – was largely taking place surreptitiously and without our awareness or much public debate. Until recently, that is. The backlash against an expanded role for gambling in society, fuelled by growing dislike of the way gambling is being promoted and increased awareness of gambling's harms and dangers, especially for the young, has been rising. It is become ever clearer that modern gambling is no ordinary commodity and should not be treated as such. The tide of gambling normalisation is turning.

Gambling is now mostly provided commercially, much of it by very large companies operating internationally. First and foremost, it is their interests which were being served by our tacit acceptance of gambling expansion. But it is the alliance of the gambling-providing industry and our governments, at the heart of what I have termed the *Gambling Establishment*, along with allies such as advisory bodies, industry-led social responsibility groups, legal advisors, advertising standards authorities, accountancy firms, third-sector organisations funded by industry, and some treatment providers and academic researchers, which is so powerful. We should no longer be led unthinkingly to accept what it has been telling us about gambling and its proper place in society.

I'll give the last word to Anna, whose addiction to Australian pokie machines we heard about in Chapter 6. She had this to say about the intense shame she had felt (Bardsley, 2013, p 14):

> As I step away from Shame, I realise that of those addicted to poker machines –
> and here I include the owners of the machines and the venues and the . . .
> government, all collecting an enormous amount of guaranteed revenue – the
> only ones visited by Shame are those who feed in the money.

We should all accept some share of the blame for the unthinking way in which gambling has been allowed to expand and put us all in the way of danger. But the harm, and the blame and shame which accompany it, are distributed very unequally. We need responsibility to be shared more fairly. We particularly need governments to face up to their responsibility and have a serious rethink about the proper place of gambling in the modern world.

REFERENCES

Adams, P. (2008). *Gambling, Freedom and Democracy*. London: Routledge.

Adams, P. (2016). *Moral Jeopardy: Risks of Accepting Money from the Alcohol, Tobacco and Gambling Industries*. Cambridge: Cambridge University Press.

Adams, P., Raeburn, J., & de Silva, K. (2009). A question of balance: prioritizing public health responses to harm from gambling. *Addiction*, 104, 688–91.

Ainslie, G. (2011). Free will as recursive self-production: does a deterministic mechanism reduce responsibility? In J. Poland & G. Graham (eds.), *Addiction and Responsibility*. Cambridge, MA: The MIT Press.

Alexius, S. (2017). Assigning responsibility for gambling-related harm: scrutinizing processes of direct and indirect consumer responsibilization of gamblers in Sweden. *Addiction Research & Theory*, 25, 462–75.

All Party Parliamentary Group on Fixed Odds Betting Terminals (APPG) (2017). Fixed odds betting terminals: assessing the impact, January.

American Gaming Association (2008). Submission to the Australian senate regarding the poker harm minimisation and harm reduction bills.

American Psychiatric Association (1980). *Diagnostic and Statistical Manual (DSM) of Mental Disorders* (3rd ed.). Washington, DC: APA.

American Psychiatric Association (2014). *Diagnostic and Statistical Manual (DSM) of Mental Disorders* (5th ed.). Washington, DC: APA.

AP News (2018). Albania to relocate casinos, betting shops to city outskirts, *www.apnews.com*, 9 October 2018, cited by Global Gambling Guidance group (G4), info@gx4.com, 25 October 2018.

Ariyabuddhiphongs, V. (2013). Problem gambling prevention: before, during and after measures. *International Journal of Mental Health and Addiction*, 11, 568–82.

Ars Technica (2018). 15 countries and one US state team up to fight gambling in video games, *arstechnica.com/gaming*, 17 September 2018, cited by Global Gambling Guidance group (G4), info@gx4.com, 27 September 2018.

Atherton, M. (2007). *Gambling*. London: Hodder & Stoughton.

Australasian Gaming Machine Manufacturers Association (2007). Submission to the New South Wales Government regarding the gaming machines act 2001.

Australian Productivity Commission (APC). (1999). *Australia's Gambling Industries*. Report No. 10. Canberra: Ausinfo.

Azmier, J. (2000). Canadian gambling behaviour and attitudes: Summary report. Canada West Foundation.

Babor, T. (2009). Alcohol research and the alcohol beverage industry: issues, concerns and conflicts of interest. *Addiction*, 104, 34–47.

Babor, T. (2016). The other side of the firewall: commentary on Livingstone & Adams 2016. *Addiction*, 111, 15–16.

Banks, J. (2014). *Online Gambling and Crime: Causes, Controls and Controversies*. Farnham, Surrey: Ashgate.

Bardsley, A. (2013). Shame. In A. Zable & T. Costello (eds.), *From Ruin to Recovery: Gamblers Share Their Stories*. www.monashlink.org.au.

Barnard, M., Kerr, J., Kinsella, K., Orford, J., Reith, G., & Wardle, H. (2013). Exploring the relationship between gambling, debt and financial management in Britain. *International Gambling Studies*, 14, 82–95.

Baumeister, R., Bratslavsky, E., Muraven, M., & Tice, D. (1998). Ego depletion: is the active self a limited resource? *Journal of Personality and Social Psychology*, 74, 1252–65.

Becoña, E., & Becoña, L. (2018). Gambling regulation in Spain. In M. Egerer, V. Marionneau, & J. Nikkinen (eds.), *Gambling Policies in European Welfare States: Current Challenges and Future Prospects*. Cham, Switzerland: Palgrave Macmillan, 83–97.

Beck, U. (1992). *The Risk Society: Towards a New Modernity*. London: Sage.

Beckert, J., & Lutter, M. (2009). The inequality of fair play: lottery gambling and social stratification in Germany. *European Sociological Review*, 25, 475–88 (cited by Sulkunen *et al.*, 2019).

Bereiter, D., & Storr, S. (2018). Gambling policies and law in Austria. In M. Egerer, V. Marionneau, & J. Nikkinen (eds.), *Gambling Policies in European Welfare States: Current Challenges and Future Prospects*. Cham, Switzerland: Palgrave Macmillan, 59–82.

Bestman, A., Thomas, S., Randle, M., Pitt, H., Daube, M., & Pettigrew, S. (2016). Shaping pathways to gambling consumption? An analysis of the promotion of gambling and non-gambling activities from gambling venues. *Addiction Research and Theory*, 24, 152–62.

Bickel, W., Miller, M., Yi, R., Kowal, B., Lindquist, D., & Pitcock, J. (2007). Behavioral and neuroeconomics of drug addiction: competing neural systems and temporal discounting processes. *Drug and Alcohol* Dependence, 90S, S85–91.

Binde, P. (2009). 'You could become a millionaire': truth, deception, and imagination in gambling advertising. In S. Kingma (ed.), *Global Gambling: Cultural Perspectives on Gambling Organizations*. New York: Routledge, 171–94.

Binde, P. (2013). Why people gamble: a model with five motivational dimensions. *International Gambling Studies*, 13, 81–97.

Binde, P. (2014). Gambling advertising: a critical research review (unpublished; cited by CAP & BCAP, 2015).

Blaszczynski, A., Collins, P., Fong, D., Ladouceur, R., Nower, L., Shaffer, H., Tavares, T., & Venisse, J. L. (2011). Responsible gambling: general principles and minimal requirements. *Journal of Gambling Studies*, 27, 565–73.

Blaszczynski, A., & Farrell, E. (1998). A case series of 44 completed gambling-related suicides. *Journal of Gambling Studies*, 14, 93–109.

Blaszczynski, A., Ladouceur, R., Nower, L., & Shaffer, H. (2008). Informed choice and gambling: principles for consumer protection. *Journal of Gambling, Business and Economics*, 2, 103–18.

Blaszczynski, A., Ladouceur, R., & Shaffer, H. (2004). A science-based framework for responsible gambling: the Reno model. *Journal of Gambling Studies*, 20, 301–17.

Borch, A. (2018). Why restrict? Seven explanations for the electronic gambling machines monopoly in Norway. In M. Egerer, V. Marionneau, & J. Nikkinen (eds.), *Gambling Policies in European Welfare States: Current Challenges and Future Prospects*. Cham, Switzerland: Palgrave Macmillan, 175–95.

Bowden-Jones, H., & Prever, F. (2017). *Gambling Disorders in Women: An International Female Perspective on Treatment and Research*. London: Routledge.

Brady, M. (2004). *Regulating Social Problems: The Pokies, the Productivity Commission and Aboriginal Communities*. Canberra: The Centre for Aboriginal Economic Policy Research, Australian National University. www.anu.edu.au.

Brenner, R., & Brenner, G. (1990). *Gambling and Speculation: A Theory, a History, and a Future of Some Human Decisions*. Cambridge: Cambridge University Press.

Bruneau, M., Guillou-Landreat, M., Challet-Bouju, G., Leboucher, J., Sauvaget, A., Caillon, J., & Grall-Bronnec, M. (2017). Gambling problems in women: French specificities. In H. Bowden-Jones & & F. Prever (eds.), *Gambling Disorders in Women: An International Female Perspective on Treatment and Research*. London: Routledge, 112–23.

Bullock, S., & Potenza, M. (2015). Pharmacological treatments. In H. Bowden-Jones & S. George (eds.), *A Clinician's Guide to Working with Problem Gamblers*. Abingdon, England: Routledge, 134–62.

CalvinAyre (2018a). Belgium's new restrictive online gambling rules close to reality, 16 January 2018, cited by Global Gambling Guidance group (G4), info@gx4.com, 21 February 2018.

CalvinAyre (2018b). Japan proposes casino entry fee of ¥2000 (US$18.50) for locals. 21 February 2018. https://calvinayre.com/2018.

Cantinotti, M., & Ladouceur, R. (2008). Harm reduction and electronic gambling machines: does this pair make a happy couple or is divorce foreseen? *Journal of Gambling* Studies, 24, 39–54.

CAP & BCAP (Committee of Advertising Practice and Broadcast Committee of Advertising Practice) (2015). CAP and BCAP gambling review: an assessment of the regulatory implications of new and emerging evidence for the UK Advertising Codes. Report prepared at the request of the Department for Culture, Media and Sport (DCMS).

Carers Trust. (2013). *The triangle of care: careers included: a guide to best practice in mental health care in England* (2nd ed.). www.carers.org.

Carrà, G., Crocamo, C., & Bebbington, P. (2017). Gambling, geographical variations and deprivation: findings from the adult psychiatric morbidity survey. *International Gambling Studies*, 17, 459–70.

Carroll, A., Rogers, B., Davidson, T., & Sims, S. (2013). *Stigma and Help-Seeking for Gambling Problems*. Canberra: Australian National University.

Casey, D. (2018). The DNA of bingo: charity and online bingo. In M. Egerer, V. Marionneau, & J. Nikkinen (eds.), *Gambling Policies in European Welfare States: Current Challenges and Future Prospects*. Cham, Switzerland: Palgrave Macmillan, 153–71.

Casey, E. (2003). Gambling and consumption: working-class women and UK national lottery play. *Journal of Consumer Culture*, 3, 245–63.

Casino News Daily (2018). A total of 29,319 Belgians excluded themselves from gambling in 2017. *casinonewsdaily.com*, 23 April 2018, cited by Global Gambling Guidance group (G4), info@gx4.com, 26 April 2018.

Casino Players Report (2017). Czech ministry of finance issues new consumer gambling protections, 31 July 2017. www.casinoplayersreport.com.

Cassidy, R., Loussouarn, C., & Pisac, A. (2013). *Fair Game: Producing Gambling Research. The Goldsmiths Report*. Goldsmiths: University of London.

Casswell, S., Quan You, R., & Huckle, T. (2011). Alcohol's harm to others: reduced wellbeing and health status for those with heavy drinkers in their lives. *Addiction*, 106, 1087–94.

Castrén, S., Basnet, S., Pankakoski, M., Ronkainen, J., Helakorpi, S., Uutela, A., & Lahti, T. (2013). An analysis of problem gambling among the Finnish working-age population: a population survey. *BMC Public Heath*, 13, 519 (cited by Sulkunen *et al.*, 2019).

Chambers, K. (2011). *Gambling for Profit: Lotteries, Gaming Machines, and Casinos in Cross-National Focus*. Toronto: University of Toronto Press (cited by Sulkunen *et al.*, 2019).

Chandler, C., & Andrews, A. (2018). *Addiction: A Biopsychosocial Perspective*. London: Sage.

Cisneros Örnberg, J., & Hettne, J. (2018). The future Swedish gambling market: challenges in law and public policies. In M. Egerer, V. Marionneau, & J. Nikkinen (eds.), *Gambling Policies in European Welfare States: Current Challenges and Future Prospects*. Cham, Switzerland: Palgrave Macmillan, 197–216.

Clapson, M. (1992). *A Bit of a Flutter: Popular Gambling and English Society, c.1823–1961*. Manchester: Manchester University Press.

Clark, L. (2015). Commentary on Cassidy, Fair game? Producing and publishing gambling research. *International Gambling* Studies, 15, 10–11.

Clark, L., Lawrence, A., Astley-Jones, F., & Gray, N. (2009). Gambling near-misses enhance motivation to gamble and recruit win-related brain circuitry. *Neuron*, 61, 481–90.

Clarke, D., Tse, S., Abbott, M., Townsend, S., Kingi, P., & Manaia, W. (2006). Key indicators of the transition from social to problem gambling. *International Journal of Mental Health and* Addiction, 4, 247–64.

Collins, D. (2014). Understanding return-to-player messages. Paper presented at the conference Harm Minimisation: Investigating Gaming Machines in Licensed Betting Offices, London, 10 December 2014.

Collins, P. (2003). *Gambling and the Public Interest*. Westport: Praeger.

Collins, P., Blaszczynski, A., Ladouceur, R., Shaffer, H., Fong, G., & Venisse, J-L. (2015). Responsible gambling: conceptual considerations. *Gaming Law Review and Economics*, 3, 594–9.

The Conversation (2018). Gambling or gaming: study shows almost half of loot boxes in video games constitute gambling, theconversation.com/gaming, 28 June 2018, cited by Global Gambling Guidance group (G4), info@gx4.com, 12 July 2018.

Copello, A., Templeton, L., Orford, J., & Velleman, R. (2010). The 5-Step method: evidence of gains for affected family members. *Drugs: Education, Prevention & Policy*, 17(S), 100–12.

Corporate Research Associates (2006). *Nova Scotia video lottery program changes impact analysis*. Halifax, Nova Scotia Gaming Corporation (cited by Sulkunen *et al.*, 2019).

Cowlishaw, S., Merkouris, S., Dowling, N., Anderson, C., Jackson, A., & Thomas, S. (2012). Psychological therapies for pathological and problem gambling. The Cochrane Library, doi:10.1002/14651858.CD008937.pub2.

Custer, R., & Milt, H. (1985). *When Luck Runs Out: Help for Compulsive Gamblers and Their Families*. New York: Facts on File.

da Cunha, D. (2010). *Singapore Places Its Bets: Casinos, Foreign Talent and Remaking a City-State*. Singapore: Straits Times Press Reference.

Daily Mail (2001). 18 July. See also Daily Mail online, 17 February 2011, I was savaged for saying my party sold its soul by letting gambling boom. I take no pride in having been proved right.

Daily Mail (2007). A busted flush: despite her wheeler-dealing, peers leave Jowell's casino plan in tatters, 29 March 2007.

Daily Mail (2018a). When will we rein in gambling sharks with blood on their hands? 25 June 2018.

Daily Mail (2018b). Italy bans advertising on all forms of gambling as part of new 'dignity decree' after populist 5-Star leader said betting destroys families, 5 July 2018. www.dailymail.co.uk/news.

Daube, M., & Stoneham, M. (2016). Gambling with interests: commentary on Livingstone and Adams 2016. *Addiction*, 111, 12–13.

Deans, E., Thomas, S., Derevensky, J., & Daube, M. (2017). The influence of marketing on the sports betting attitudes and consumption behaviours of young men: implications for harm reduction and prevention strategies. *Harm Reduction Journal*, 14, 1–12.

Değirmencioğlu, S., & Walker, C. (eds.). (2015). *Social and Psychological Dimensions of Personal Debt and the Debt Industry*. Basingstoke, Hampshire: Palgrave Macmillan.

Delfabbro, P. (2014). A view from the machines research oversight panel. Paper presented at the Responsible Gambling Trust conference, Harm Minimisation: Investigating Gaming Machines in Licensed Betting Offices. London, 10 December 2014.

Delfabbro, P., Borgas, M., & King, D. (2011). Venue staff knowledge of their patrons' gambling and problem gambling. *Journal of Gambling Studies*, published online 1 June 2011, doi:10.1007/s10899-011-9252-2.

Denzin, N. (1987). *The Alcoholic Self*. Thousand Islands: Sage.

Department for Culture, Media and Sport (DCMS) (2002). *A Safe Bet for Success: Modernising Britain's Gambling Laws*. London: The Stationery Office.

Department for Digital, Culture, Media and Sport (2017a). Consultation on proposals for changes to gaming machines and social responsibility measures, 31 October 2017. www.gov.uk/government/consultations.

Department for Digital, Culture, Media and Sport (2017b). Responses to the call for evidence: review of gaming machines and social responsibility measures, 31 October 2017. www.gov.uk/government/consultations.

Derevensky, J., Sklar, A., Gupta, R., & Messerlain, C. (2010). An empirical study examining the impact of gambling advertisements on adolescent gambling attitudes and behaviors. *International Journal of Mental Health and Addiction*, 10, 21–34.

Dickerson, M. (1990). Gambling: the psychology of a non-drug compulsion. *Drug and Alcohol Review*, 9, 187–99.

Dickerson, M., & O'Connor, J. (2006). *Gambling as an Addictive Behaviour: Impaired Control, Harm Minimisation, Treatment and Prevention*. Cambridge: Cambridge University Press.

Dickson-Gillespie, L., Rugle, L., Rosenthal, R., & Fong, T. (2008). Preventing the incidence and harm of gambling problems. *Journal of Primary Prevention*, 29, 37–55.

Dixon, D. (1991). *From Prohibition to Regulation: Bookmaking, Anti-Gambling and the Law*. Oxford: Clarendon Press.

Dixon, M., Larche, C., Stange, M., & Fugelsang, J. (2018b). Near-misses and stop buttons in slot machine play: an investigation of how they affect players and may foster erroneous cognitions. *Journal of Gambling Studies*, 34, 161–80.

Dixon, M., Stange, M., Larche, C., & Graydon, C. (2018a). Dark flow, depression and multi-line slot machine play. *Journal of Gambling Studies*, 34, 73–84.

Dostoevsky, F. (1866). *The Gambler*. Moscow: Fyodor Stellovsky (Penguin Random House, 2003).

Dowling, N., Suomi, A., Jackson, A., Lavis, T., Patford, J., Cockman, S., Thomas, S., Bellringer, M., Koziol-Mclain, J., Battersby, M., Harvey, P., & Abbott, M. (2016). Problem gambling and intimate partner violence: a systematic review and meta-analysis. *Trauma, Violence and Abuse*, 17, 43–61.

The Drum (2014). William Hill, Ladbrokes and Paddy Power to tighten responsible-gambling messaging, 30 December 2014. www.thedrum.com/news.

Eadington, W. (2008). Gambling Policy in European Union: Monopolies, market access, economic rents, and competitive pressures among gaming sectors in the member states. In T. Coryn, C. Fijnaut, & A. Littler (eds.), *The Economic Aspects of Gambling Regulation: EU and US Perspectives*. Leiden: Martinus Nijhoff, 71–90.

The Economist (2017). Australians spend more on gambling than people anyone else; the industry spends a fair bit on lobbying too, 16 March 2017, cited by Global Gambling Guidance group (G4), info@gx4.com, 11 May 2017.

European Monitoring Centre for Drugs and Drug Addiction (2018). European drug report 2018: Trends and developments. EMCDDA, June 2018.

Excell, D., & Bobashev, G. (2014). Predicting problem gamblers: analysis of industry data. Paper presented at the responsible gambling trust conference, harm minimisation: investigating gaming machines in licensed betting offices. London, 10 December 2014.

Financial Times (2017). How UK beat the odds to win at online gambling, 12 August 2017. www.ft.com.

Friedman, B. (2000). *Designing Casinos to Dominate the Competition*. Reno, NV: Institute for the Study of Gambling and Commercial Gaming (cited by Schüll, 2012).

Gainsbury, S. (2012). *Internet Gambling: Current Research Findings and Implications*. New York: Springer.

Gainsbury, S. (2014). Review of self-exclusion from gambling venues as an intervention for problem gambling. *Journal of Gambling Studies*, 30, 229–51.

Gainsbury, S., Blankers, M., Wilkinson, C., Schelleman-Offermans, K., & Cousijn, J. (2014). Recommendations for international gambling harm-minimisation guidelines: comparison with effective public health policy. *Journal of Gambling Studies*, 30, 771–88.

Gainsbury, S., Delfabbro, P., King, D., & Hing, N. (2015). An exploratory study of gambling operators' use of social media and the latent messages conveyed. *Journal of Gambling Studies*, published online 3 February 2015, doi:10.1007/s10899-015-9525-2.

GambleAware (2017a). Remote gambling research: interim report on phase II. about. gambleaware.org/research.

GambleAware (2017b). Statistics for gambling treatment in Great Britain 2016–2017 from the data reporting framework. about.gambleaware.org

Gambling (Licensing and Advertising) Act (2014). www.legislation.gov.uk/ukpga/2014.

Gambling Commission (2015). Strengthening social responsibility: amendments to the social responsibility provisions in the LCCP and to Remote technical standards: summary of key changes, February 2015. www.gamblingcommission.gov.uk.

Gambling Commission (2017). Fairer and safer gambling, CEO keynote speech, Raising standards conference, 21 November 2017, Gambling Commission e-bulletin, 23 November 2017.

Gambling Commission (2018a). William Hill to pay £6.2m penalty package for systemic social responsibility and money laundering failures, Gambling Commission e-bulletin, 26 February 2018.

Gambling Commission (2018b). 32Red to pay £2m penalty package for failing to protect customer. Gambling Commission website. www.gamblingcommission.gov.uk/news.

Gambling Commission (2019a). Industry statistics, appendix 2. April 2015 to March 2018. Gambling Commission website. www.gamblingcommission.gov.uk.

Gambling Commission (2019b). Gambling participation in 2018: behaviour, awareness and attitudes, Annual Report February 2019. Gambling Commission website. www.gambling commission.gov.uk.

Gambling Review Body (2001). *Gambling Review Report*. Department for Culture, Media and Sport. Norwich: HMSO.

Gaming Board (2000). *Report of the Gaming Board for Great Britain 1999/2000*. London: HMSO.

Gavriel-Fried, B. (2015). Attitudes of Jewish Israeli adults towards gambling. *International Gambling Studies*, 15, 196–211.

George, S., Kallilvayalil, R., & Jaisoorya, T. (2014). Gambling addiction in India: should psychiatrists care? *Indian Journal of Psychiatry*, 56, 111–12.

Gidluck, L. (2016). A global comparison of how governments regulate, operate and benefit from state lotteries. All Bets are Off Conference, Canterbury, England, 24 June 2016 (cited by Sulkunen *et al.*, 2019).

Glasby, J. (2011). From evidence-based to knowledge-based policy and practice. In J. Glasby (ed.), *Evidence, Policy and Practice: Critical Perspectives in Health and Social Care*. Bristol: The Policy Press, 85–98.

Goh, C. (2017). The psychology of gaming and gambling. Unpublished Doctor of Clinical Psychology thesis, University of Birmingham.

Goh, E., Ng, V., & Yeoh, B. (2016). The family exclusion order as a harm-minimisation measure for casino gambling: the case of Singapore. *International Gambling Studies*, 16, 373–90.

Goodman, R. (1995). *The Luck Business: The Devastating Consequences and Broken Promises of America's Gambling Explosion*. New York: The Free Press.

Goodwin, B., Browne, M., Rockloff, M., & Rose, J. (2017). A typical problem gambler affects six others. *International Gambling Studies*, 17, 276–89.

Griffiths, M. (1993). Fruit machine addiction in adolescents: a case study. *Journal of Gambling Studies*, 9, 387–99.

Griffiths, M. (2010). The role of parents in the development of gambling behaviour in adolescents. *Education and Health*, 28, 51–54.

Grinols, E. (2003). Cutting the cards and craps: right thinking about gambling economics. In G. Reith (ed.), *Gambling: Who Wins? Who Loses?* New York: Prometheus, 67–87.

Grun, L., & McKeigue, P. (2000). Prevalence of excessive gambling before and after introduction of a national lottery in the United Kingdom: another example of the single distribution theory. *Addiction*, 95, 959–66.

The Guardian (2001). Big win for punters, 5 October 2001. www.theguardian.com/money.

The Guardian (2017). UK gambling industry now takes £14bn a year from punters, 31 August 2017. www.theguardian.com.

The Guardian (2018a). 'Easy trap to fall into': why video-game loot boxes need regulation, *www.theguardian.com*, 29 May 2018, cited by Global Gambling Guidance group (G4), info@gx4.com, 26 June 2018.

The Guardian (2018b). Sports minister resigns over delay to gambling curb, 1 November 2018.

Häfeli, J. (2014). Paper presented at Excessive gambling: prevention and harm reduction, a conference held at the University of Neuchâtel, Switzerland, 15–17 January 2014.

Häfeli, J., & Schneider, C. (2006). The early detection of problem gamblers in casinos: a new screening instrument. Paper presented at the Asian Pacific Gambling Conference, Hong Kong (cited by Delfabbro *et al.*, 2011).

Hancock, L. (2016). Fine-tuning Livingstone and Adams' ethical principles for integrity in gambling research: commentary on Livingstone and Adams 2016. *Addiction*, 111, 13–15.

Hancock, L., & Orford, J. (2014). FOBTs – beyond regulation? *New Statesman*, 16–22 May 2014.

Hancock, L., & Smith, G. (2017). Critiquing the Reno model I-IV international influence on regulators and governments (2004–2015) – the distorted reality of 'responsible gambling'.

International Journal of Mental Health and Addiction, published online 24 April 2017, doi:10.1007/s11469-017-9746-y.

Harrigan, K., & Dixon, M. (2009). PAR sheets, probabilities, and slot machine play: implications for problem and non-problem gambling. *Journal of Gambling Issues*, 23, 81–110.

Harrigan, K., & Dixon, M. (2010). Government sanctioned 'tight' and 'loose' slot machines: how having multiple versions of the same slot machine game may impact problem gambling. *Journal of Gambling Studies*, 26, 159–74.

Hing, N., Lamont, M., Vitartas, P., & Fink, E. (2015). Sports-embedded gambling promotions: a study of exposure, sports betting intention and problem gambling amongst adults. *International Journal of Mental Health and Addiction*, 13, 115–35.

Hing, N., Nuske, E., & Breen, H. (2017). A review of research into problem gambling amongst Australian women. In H. Bowden-Jones & F. Prever (eds.), *Gambling Disorders in Women: An International Female Perspective on Treatment and Research*. London: Routledge, 235–46.

Hing, N., Nuske, E., Gainsbury, S., & Russell, A. (2016). Perceived stigma and self-stigma of problem gambling: perspectives of people with gambling problems. *International Gambling Studies*, 16, 31–48.

Hogarth, L. (2019). Controlled and automatic learning processes in addiction. In H. Pickard & S. Ahmed (eds.), *The Routledge Handbook of Philosophy and Science of Addiction*. London: Routledge, 325–38.

Horváth, C., & Paap, R. (2012). The effects of recessions on gambling expenditures. *Journal of Gambling Studies*, 28, 703–17 (cited by Sulkunen *et al.*, 2019).

House of Commons, Culture, Media and Sport Committee (2012). The gambling act 2005: a bet worth taking? 12 July 2012.

iGB Affiliate (2019). Swedish self-exclusion scheme hits 10.000 sign-ups, *igbaffiliate*, 8 January 2019, cited by Global Gambling Guidance group (G4), info@gx4.com, 29 January 2019.

iGaming Business (2019a). GamStop says ID changes will enhance self-exclusion service, 14 January 2019, cited by Global Gambling Guidance group (G4), info@gx4.com, 29 January 2019.

iGaming Business (2019b). Gambling operators face new UK advertising controls, 13 February 2019. igamingbusiness.com/news.

Independent (2018). Bet365 boss Denise Coates' pay rises to 'eye-watering' £265m, 21 November 2018. www.independent.co.uk/news.

Ingle, P., Marotta, J., McMillan, G., & Wisdom, J. (2008). Significant others and gambling treatment outcome. *Journal of Gambling Studies*, 24, 381–92.

Institute for Public Policy Research (IPPR) (2016). *Cards on the Table: The Cost to Government of Problem Gambling in Great Britain*. London: IPPR.

International Business Times (2018). Australia to commence stronger gambling advertising restrictions from March 30. www.ibtimes.com.au, 19 March 2018, cited by Global Gambling Guidance group (G4), info@gx4.com, 28 March 2018.

Ipsos Mori (2009). British survey of children, the national lottery and gambling 2008–09: report of a quantitative survey (cited by Griffiths, 2010).

Jacobs, D., Marston, A., Singer, R., Widsman, K., Little, T., & Veizades, J. (1989). Children of problem gamblers. *Journal of Gambling Behavious*, 5, 261–8.

James, W. (1891). *The Principles of Psychology, Volume 1*. London: Macmillan.

Jiménez-Murcia, S., Tremblay, J., Stinchfield, R. *et al.* (18 others). (2016). The involvement of a concerned significant other in gambling disorder treatment outcome. *Journal of Gambling Behavior*, 33, 937–53.

Jones, C. (2017). Football and the normalisation of gambling. Paper presented at GambleAware 5th Harm Minimisation Conference, London, 6–7 December 2017.

Jones, C., Pinder, R., & Robinson, G. (2019). Gambling sponsorship and advertising in British football: a critical account. *Sport, Ethics and Philosophy*, published online 27 February 2019. doi:10.1080/17511321.2019.1582558.

Jones, O. (2015). *The Establishment and How They Get Away with It*. London: Penguin Books.

Karlsson, A., & Håkansson, A. (2018). Gambling disorder, increased mortality, suicidality, and associated comorbidity: a longitudinal nationwide register study. *Journal of Behavioural Addictions*, 7, 1091–9.

Karter, L. (2013). *Women and Problem Gambling: Therapeutic Insights into Understanding Addiction and Treatment*. London: Routledge.

Kelly, T. (2013). *Red Card: The Soccer Star Who Lost It All to Gambling*. Chichester, England: Mereo.

King, D., & Delfabbro, P. (2018). Predatory monetisation schemes in video games (e.g. 'loot boxes') and internet gambling disorder. Editorial, *Addiction*, 113, 1967–9.

King, D., Delfabbro, P., & Griffiths, M. (2009). The convergence of gambling and digital media: implications for gambling in young people. *Journal of Gambling Studies*, 26, 175–87.

Kingma, S. (2004). Gambling and the risk society: the liberalisation and legitimation crisis of gambling in the Netherlands. *International Gambling Studies*, 4, 47–67 (cited by Sulkunen *et al.*, 2019).

Kindt, J. (2012). *The Gambling Threat to National and Homeland Security: Internet Gambling*. Research Editors Doctoral Directorate on Gambling. Buffalo, NY: William S Hein.

Knapp, T. (1997). Behaviorism and public policy: BF Skinner's views on gambling. *Behavior and Social Issues*, 7, 129–39.

Konietzny, J. (2017). No risk, no fun: implications for positioning of online casinos. *International Gambling Studies*, 17, 144–59.

Kotter, R., Kräplin, A., & Bühringer, G. (2018). Casino self- or forced excluders' gambling behaviour before and after exclusion. *Journal of Gambling Studies*, 34, 597–612.

Labour Party (2017). Labour party review of problem gambling and its treatment. www.tom-watson.com/gambling.

LaBrie, R., LaPlante, D., Nelson, S., Schumann, A., & Shaffer, H. (2007). Assessing the playing field: a prospective longitudinal study of internet sports gambling behavior. *Journal of Gambling Studies*, 23, 347–62.

Ladouceur, R., Boisvert, J., Pepin, M., Lorangere, M., & Sylvain, C. (1994). Social cost of pathological gambling. *Journal of Gambling Studies*, 10, 399–409.

Langer, E., & Roth, J. (1975). Heads I win, tails it's chance: the illusion of control as a function of the sequence of outcomes in a purely chance task. *Journal of Personality and Social Psychology*, 32, 951–5.

Langham, E., Thorne, H., Browne, M., Donaldson, P., Rose, J., & Rockloff, M. (2016). Understanding gambling related harm: a proposed definition, conceptual framework, and taxonomy of harms. *BMC Public Health*, 16, 80.

Larcombe, J. (2014). *Tails I Lose: The Compulsive Gambler Who Lost His Shirt for Good*. Oxford: Lion Books.

Leino, T., Torsheim, T., Pallesen, S., Blaszczynski, A., Sagoe, D., & Molde, H. (2016). An empirical real-world study of losses disguised as wins in electronic gambling machines. *International Gambling Studies*, 16, 470–80.

Lepper, J., & Creigh-Tyte, S. (2013). The national lottery. In L. Vaughan-Williams & D. Siegel (eds.), *The Oxford Handbook of the Economics of Gambling*. New York: Oxford University Press, 611–36 (cited by Sulkunen *et al.*, 2019).

Lesieur, H. (1984). *The Chase: The Career of the Compulsive Gambler*. Rochester, VT: Schenkman.

Levy, N. (2006). Autonomy and addiction. *Canadian Journal of Philosophy*, 36, 427–47.

Lewis, M. (2015). *The Biology of Desire: Why Addiction Is Not a Disease*. Melbourne: Scribe.

Lim, M., Bowden-Jones, H., Salinas, M., Price, J., Goodwin, G., Geddes, J., & Rogers, R. (2016). The experience of gambling problems in British professional footballers: a preliminary qualitative study. *Addiction Research and Theory*, 25, 129–38.

Livingstone, C., & Adams, P. (2016). Clear principles are needed for integrity in gambling research. *Addiction*, 111, 5–10.

Livingstone, C., & Woolley, R. (2007). Risky business: a few provocations on the regulation of electronic gaming machines. *International Gambling Studies*, 7, 361–76.

Loer, K. (2018). Gambling and doing good? On the relationship between gambling regulations and welfare services in Germany. In M. Egerer, V. Marionneau, & J. Nikkinen (eds.), *Gambling Policies in European Welfare States: Current Challenges and Future Prospects*. Cham, Switzerland: Palgrave Macmillan, 101–18.

Lopez-Gonzalez, H., & Griffiths, M. (2016). Is European gambling regulation adequately addressing in-play betting advertising? *Gaming Law Review and Economics*, 20, 495–503.

Lopez-Gonzalez, H., Estévez, A., & Griffiths, M. (2018a). Controlling the illusion of control: a grounded theory of sports betting advertising in the UK. *International Gambling Studies*, 18, 39–55.

Lopez-Gonzalez, H., & Griffiths, M. (2018b). Betting, forex trading and fantasy gaming sponsorships: a responsible gambling inquiry into the gamblification of English football. *International Journal of Mental Health and Addiction*, 16, 404–19.

Lopez-Gonzalez, H., Guerrero-Solé, F., & Griffiths, M. (2018c). A content analysis of how 'normal' sports betting behaviour is represented in gambling advertising. *Addiction Research & Theory*, 26, 238–47.

Lorenz, V. (1987). Family dynamics of pathological gamblers. In T. Galski (ed.), *The Handbook of Pathological Gambling*. Springfield, IL: Charles C. Thomas.

Lukes, S. (2005). *Power: A Radical View*. Basingstoke, Hampshire: Palgrave Macmillan.

MacLaren, V. (2015). Video lottery is the most harmful form of gambling in Canada. *Journal of Gambling Studies*, published online 2 August 2015, doi:10.1007/s10899-015-9560-z.

Madge, C., & Harrisson, T. (1939). *Britain by Mass Observation*. Harmondsworth: Penguin.

Marionneau, V., & Berret, S. (2018). Gambling for the state: the collection and redistribution of gambling proceeds in France. In M. Egerer, V. Marionneau, & J. Nikkinen (eds.), *Gambling Policies in European Welfare States: Current Challenges and Future Prospects*. Cham, Switzerland: Palgrave Macmillan, 17–35.

Marionneau, V., Nikkinen, J., & Egerer, M. (2018). Conclusions: contradictions in promoting gambling for good causes. In M. Egerer, V. Marionneau, & J. Nikkinen (eds.), *Gambling Policies in European Welfare States: Current Challenges and Future Prospects*. Cham. Switzerland: Palgrave Macmillan, 297–314.

Markham, F., & Young, M. (2014a). 'Big gambling': the rise of the global industry-state gambling complex. *Addiction Research and Theory*, 23, 1–4.

Markham, F., & Young, M. (2014b). Who wins from 'Big Gambling' in Australia? *The Conversation*, 5 March 2014. https://theconversation.co (cited by Sulkunen *et al.*, 2019).

Marshall, D., & Baker, R. (2001). Clubs, spades, diamonds and disadvantage: the geography of electronic gambling machines in Melbourne. *Australian Geographical Studies*, 39, 17–33.

Mathews, M., & Volberg, R. (2013). Impact of problem gambling on financial, emotional and social well-being of Singaporean families. *International Gambling Studies*, 13, 127–140.

Matuszewski, E. (2014). Daily fantasy cites buy sponsorship to build on $1 billion fees. *Bloomberg*, 18 December 2014. Online www.bloomberg.com/news/articles/2014-12-18 (cited by Sulkunen *et al.*, 2019).

McCambridge, J., Mialon, M., & Hawkins, B. (2018). Alcohol industry involvement in policy making: a systematic review. *Addiction,* published online 15 March 2018, doi:10.1111/add.14216.

McComb, J., Lee, B., & Sprenkle, D. (2009). Conceptualizing and treating problem gambling as a family issue. *Journal of Marital and Family Therapy,* 35, 415–31.

McCormack, A., & Griffiths, M. (2012). Motivating and inhibiting factors in online gambling behaviour: a grounded theory study. *International Journal of Mental Health and Addiction,* 10, 39–53.

McMillen, J. (2003). From local to global gambling cultures. In G. Reith (ed.), *Gambling: Who Wins? Who Loses?* New York: Prometheus, 49–63.

McMullan, J., & Kervin, M. (2012). Selling internet gambling: advertising, new media and the content of poker promotion. *International Journal of Mental Health and Addiction,* 10, 622–45.

Messerlian, C., Derevensky, J., & Gupta, R. (2004). A public health perspective for youth gambling. *International Gambling Studies,* 4, 147–60.

Meyer, G., & Stadler, M. (1999). Criminal behaviour associated with pathological gambling. *Journal of Gambling Studies,* 15, 29–43.

Miers, D. (2004). *Regulating Commercial Gambling: Past, Present, and Future.* Oxford: Oxford University Press.

Miller, H., Thomas, S., Smith, K., & Robinson, P. (2016). Surveillance, responsibility and control: an analysis of government and industry discourses about 'problem' and 'responsible' gambling. *Addiction Research and Theory,* 24, 163–76.

Molinaro, S., Canale, N., Vienno, A., Lenzi, M., Siciliano, V., Gori, M., & Santinello, M. (2014). Country- and individual-level determinants of probable problematic gambling in adolescence: a multi-level cross-national comparison. *Addiction,* 109, 2089–97.

Monaghan, M. (2011). *Evidence Versus Politics: Exploiting Research in UK Drug Policy Making.* Bristol: Policy Press.

Monaghan, S., Derevensky, J., & Sklar, A. (2008). Impact of gambling advertisements and marketing on children and adolescents: policy recommendations to minimise harm. *Journal of Gambling Issues,* 22, 252–74 (cited by CAP & BCAP, 2015).

Murphy, D., & Smart, G. (2019). Mechanistic models for understanding addiction as a behavioural disorder. In H. Pickard & S. Ahmed (eds.), *The Routledge Handbook of Philosophy and Science of Addiction.* London: Routledge, 315–24.

National Housing and Town Planning Council. (1988). *The Use of the Fruit Machine.* London: The National Council on Gambling (cited by Griffiths, M., 1990, Addiction to fruit machines: a preliminary study among young males. *Journal of Gambling Studies,* 6, 113–26).

National Opinion Poll (UK) (2003).

National Research Council, National Academy of Sciences, Committee on the Social and Economic Impact of Pathological Gambling (1999). *Pathological Gambling: A Critical Review.* Washington, DC: National Academy Press.

Newall, P. (2015). How bookies make your money. *Judgement and Decision Making,* 10, 225–31.

Newall, P. (2017). Behavioral complexity of British gambling advertising. *Addiction Research and Theory,* 25, 505–11.

The New York Times (2018). Australians are the world's biggest gambling losers, and some seek action, 4 April 2018, cited by Global Gambling Guidance group (G4). info@gx4.com, 26 April 2018.

Nippon.com (2018). Gambling addiction in the land of pachinko. www.nippon.com, 4 January 2018, cited by Global Gambling Guidance group (G4), info@gx4.com, 21 February 2018.

O'Connor, P. (2019). Our stories, our knowledge: the importance of addicts' epistemic authority in treatment. In H. Pickard & S. Ahmed (eds.), *The Routledge Handbook of Philosophy and Science of Addiction*. London: Routledge, 431–9.

Ofcom (2013). Trends in advertising activity – gambling. www.ofcom.org.uk/data.

Online Casino City (2015). New Jersey division of gaming enforcement gives affiliates 150 days to comply in order to obtain license, 10 June 2015. online.casinocity.com.

Orford, J. (1985). *Excessive Appetites: A Psychological View of Addictions*. Chichester, England: Wiley, 2nd ed., 2001.

Orford, J. (2008). *Community Psychology: Challenges, Controversies and Emerging Consensus*. Chichester, England: Wiley.

Orford, J. (2011). *An Unsafe Bet? The Dangerous Rise of Gambling and the Debate We Should be Having*. Chichester, England: Wiley-Blackwell.

Orford, J. (2012). *Addiction Dilemmas: Family Experiences in Literature and Research and Their Lessons for Practice*. Chichester, England: Wiley-Blackwell.

Orford, J. (2013). *Power, Powerlessness and Addiction*. Cambridge: Cambridge University Press.

Orford, J. (2018). Problem gambling: a shared responsibility: a summary of the first 500 comments submitted to the gambling watch UK website. Paper presented at Gambling addiction: science, independence, transparency: 4th international multidisciplinary symposium, University of Fribourg, Switzerland, 27–29 June 2018.

Orford, J., Cousins, J., Smith, N., & Bowden-Jones, H. (2017). Stress, strain, coping and social support for affected family members attending the national problem gambling clinic, London. *International Gambling Studies*, 17, 259–75.

Orford, J., Griffiths, M., Wardle, H., Sproston, K., & Erens, B. (2009). Negative public attitudes towards gambling: findings from the 2007 British gambling prevalence survey using a new attitude scale. *International Gambling Studies*, 9, 39–54.

Orford, J., Sproston, K., Erens, B., White, C., & Mitchell, L. (2003). *Gambling and Problem Gambling in Britain*. Hove, England: Brunner-Routledge.

Orford, J., Wardle, H., & Griffiths, M. (2013). What proportion of gambling is problem gambling? Estimates from the 2010 British gambling prevalence survey. *International Gambling Studies*, 13, 4–18.

Orford, J., Wardle, H., Griffiths, M., Sproston, K., & Erens, B. (2010). The role of social factors in gambling: evidence from the 2007 British Gambling Prevalence Survey. *Community, Work and Family*, 13, 257–71.

Pearce, J., Mason, K., Hiscock, R., & Day, P. (2008). A national study of neighbourhood access to gambling opportunities and individual gambling behavior. *Journal of Epidemiology and Community Health*, 62, 862–8.

Petry, N. (2005). *Pathological Gambling: Etiology, Comorbidity, and Treatment*. Washington DC: American Psychological Association.

Pickard, H., & Ahmed, S. (eds.). (2019). *The Routledge Handbook of Philosophy and Science of Addiction*. London: Routledge.

Prever, F., & Locati, V. (2017). Female gambling in Italy. In H. Bowden-Jones & F. Prever (eds.), *Gambling Disorders in Women: An International Female Perspective on Treatment and Research*. London: Routledge, 125–40.

Reith, G. (1999). *The Age of Chance: Gambling in Western Culture*. London: Routledge.

Reith, G., & Dobbie, F. (2012). Lost in the games: narratives of addiction and identity in recovery from problem gambling. *Addiction Research and Theory*, 20, 511–21.

Responsible Gambling Strategy Board (2016). The national responsible gambling strategy 2016–17 to 2018–19. London RGSB, 11 April 2016.

Rintoul, A., Livingstone, C., Mellor, A., & Jolley, D. (2013). Modelling vulnerability to gambling related harm: how disadvantage predicts gambling losses. *Addiction Research and Theory*, 21, 329–38.

Robinson, T. & Berridge, K. (2000). The psychology and neurobiology of addiction: an incentive sensitization view. *Addiction*, 95, 91–117.

Rolando, S., & Scavarda, S. (2018). Italian gambling regulation: justifications and counter-arguments. In M. Egerer, V. Marionneau, & J. Nikkinen (eds.), *Gambling Policies in European Welfare States: Current Challenges and Future Prospects*. Cham, Switzerland: Palgrave Macmillan, 37–57.

Room, R. (2016). Integrity without extinction: paths forward for gambling research: commentary on Livingstone & Adams 2016. *Addiction*, 111, 11–12.

Rose, I. (1991). The rise and fall of the third wave: gambling will be outlawed in forty years. In W. Eadington & J. Cornelius (eds.), *Gambling and Public Policy: International Perspectives*. Reno, Nevada: University of Nevada.

Ross, D., Sharp, C., Vuchinich, R., & Spurrett, D. (2008). *Midbrain Mutiny: The Picoeconomics and Neuroeconomics of Disordered Gambling. Economic Theory and Cognitive Science*. Cambridge, MA: The MIT Press.

Russell, J., & Greenhalgh, T. (2011). Policy making through a rhetorical lens. In J. Glasby (ed.), *Evidence, Policy and Practice: Critical Perspectives in Health and Social Care*. Bristol: Policy Press, 49–70.

Sallaz, J. (2009). Gambling with development: comparing casino gambling legalization in South Africa with Indian gambling in California. In S. Kingma (ed.), *Global Gambling: Cultural Perspectives on Gambling Organizations*. New York: Routledge, 66–91.

Salonen, A., Castrén, S., Raisamo, S., Orford, J., Alho, H., & Lahti, T. (2014). Attitudes towards gambling in Finland: a cross-sectional population study. *BMC Public Health*, 14, 982.

Sani, A., & Zumwald, C. (2017). Effectiveness of self-exclusion: the experience of female gamblers in three Swiss casinos. In H. Bowden-Jones & F. Prever (eds.), *Gambling Disorders in Women: An International Female Perspective on Treatment and Research*. London: Routledge, 162–72.

Savell, E., Fooks, G., & Gilmour, A. (2016). How does the alcohol industry attempt to influence marketing regulations? A systematic review. *Addiction*, 111, 18–32.

Schüll, N. (2012). *Addiction by Design: Machine Gambling in Las Vegas*. Princeton: Princeton University Press.

Schwartz, D. (2006). *Roll the Bones: The History of Gambling*. New York: Gotham Books (cited by Sulkunen *et al.*, 2019).

Shaffer, H., & LaPlante, D. (2013). Considering a critique of pathological gambling prevalence research. *Addiction Research and Theory*, 21, 12–14.

Sharman, S., Dreyer, J., Clark, L., & Bowden-Jones, H. (2016). Down and out in London: addictive behaviors in homelessness. *Journal of Behavioral Addictions*, 5, 318–24.

Singer, M. (2008). *Drugging the Poor: Legal and Illegal Drugs and Social Inequality*. Long Grove, IL: Waveland Press.

Skidelsky, R., & Skidelsky, E. (2013). *How Much Is Enough? Money and the Good Life*. London: Penguin Books.

Spenwyn, J., Barrett, D., & Griffiths, M. (2010). The role of light and music in gambling behaviour: an empirical pilot study. *International Journal of Mental Health and Addiction*, 8, 107–18.

Stiglitz, J. (2013). *The Price of Inequality*. London: Penguin Books.

Stringman, C. (2017). *Win, Lose, Repeat: My Life as a Gambler, from Coin Pushers to Financial Spread-Betting*. London: Ortus (Free Association Books).

Sulkunen, P., Babor, T., Cisneros Örnberg, J., Egerer, M., Hellman, M., Livingstone, C., Marionneau, V., Nikkinen, J., Orford, J., Room, R., & Rossow, I. (2019). *Gambling: Setting Limits: Gambling, Science and Public Policy*. Oxford: Oxford University Press.

Szczyrba, Z., Mravčík, V., Fiedor, D., Černy, J., & Smolová, I. (2015). Gambling in the Czech Republic. *Addiction*, 110, 1076–81.

Tammi, T., Castrén, S., & Lintonen, T. (2015). Gambling in Finland: problem gambling in the context of a national monopoly in the European Union. *Addiction*, 110, 746–50.

Tanner, J., Drawson, A., Mushquash, C., Mushquash, A., & Mazmanian, D. (2017). Harm reduction in gambling: a systematic review of industry strategies, *Addiction Research and Theory*, 25, 485–94.

Tavares, H. (2014). Gambling in Brazil: a call for an open debate. *Addiction*, 109, 1972–6.

Tekin, Ş. (2019). Brain mechanisms and the disease model of addiction: is it the whole story of the addicted self? A philosophical-skeptical perspective. In H. Pickard & S. Ahmed (eds.), *The Routledge Handbook of Philosophy and Science of Addiction*. London: Routledge, 401–10.

The Telegraph (2010). David Cameron warns lobbying is next political scandal, 8 February 2010. www.telegraph.co.uk/news.

The Telegraph (2019). Gambling firms face compulsory levy unless they increase cash to treat addicts, says minister, 12 March 2019. www.telegraph.co.uk./politics.

Templeton, J., Dixon, M., Harrigan, K., & Fugelsang, J. (2014). Upping the reinforcement rate by playing the maximum lines in multi-line slot machine play. *Journal of Gambling Studies*, 31, 949–64.

Tepperman, L. (2009). *Betting Their Lives: The Close Relations of Problem Gamblers*. Don Mills, Ontario: Oxford University Press.

Thomas, S., Lewis, S., McLeod, C., & Haycock, J. (2012). 'They are working every angle': a qualitative study of Australian adults' attitudes towards, and interactions with, gambling industry marketing strategies. *International Gambling Studies*, 12, 111–27.

The Times (2016). Doctors prescribe drugs to tackle Britain's gambling epidemic, 17 February 2016.

Toufiq, J. (2018). Public health issues related to gambling within countries affiliated to the MedNET co-operation network. Paper presented at Gambling addiction: science, independence, transparency: 4th international multidisciplinary symposium, University of Fribourg, Switzerland, 27–29 June 2018.

Tu, D., Gray, R., & Walton, D. (2014). Household experience of gambling-related harm by socio-economic deprivation in New Zealand: increases in inequality between 2008 and 2012. *International Gambling Studies*, 14, 330–44 (cited by Sulkunen *et al.*, 2019).

Turner, N. (2011). Volatility, house edge and prize structure of gambling games. *Journal of Gambling Studies*, 27, 607–23.

Valverde, M. (1998). *Diseases of the Will: Alcohol and the Dilemmas of Freedom*. Cambridge: Cambridge University Press.

Vasiliev, P., & Bernhard, B. (2012). Prohibitions and policy in the global gambling industry: a genealogy and media content analysis of gaming restrictions in contemporary Russia. *UNLV Gaming Research & Review Journal*, 15, 71–86 (cited by Sulkunen *et al.*, 2019).

Velleman, R., Cousins, J., & Orford, J. (2015). Effects of gambling on the family. In H. Bowden-Jones & S. George (eds.), *A Clinician's Guide to Working with Problem Gamblers*. London: Royal College of Psychiatrists, 90–103.

Venturi, R., Izenour, S., & Brown, D. (1972). *Learning from Las Vegas*. Cambridge, MA: MIT Press (cited by Schüll, 2012).

Verbiest, T. (2007). French and Belgian views of the European Gambling Regulation. In A. Littler & C. Fijnaut (eds.), *The Regulation of Gambling: European and National Perspectives*. Leiden: Martinus Nijhoff, 127–59.

Vitaro, F., Wanner, B., Brendgen, M., & Tremblay, R. (2008). Offspring of parents with gambling problems: adjustment problems and explanatory mechanisms. *Journal of Gambling Studies*, 24, 535–53.

The Waikato Times (1997). The casino experience, 14 June 1997 (cited by Adams, 2008).

Ward, A. (2012). The role of host responsibility at Sky City Auckland: a practical perspective on identifying potential and problem gamblers. Paper presented at the 4th international gambling conference 2012: shaping the future of gambling – positive change through policy, action and research, Auckland, New Zealand, 22–24 February 2012.

Wardle, H. (2014). Identifying problem gambling: findings from a survey of loyalty card customers. Paper presented at the Responsible Gambling Trust conference, Harm Minimisation: Investigating Gaming Machines in Licensed Betting Offices. London, 10 December 2014.

Wardle, H. (2017). The 're-feminisation' of gambling: social, cultural and historical insights into female gambling behaviour in Great Britain. In H. Bowden-Jones & F. Prever (eds.), *Gambling Disorders in Women: An International Female Perspective on Treatment and Research.* London: Routledge, 173–86.

Wardle, H., Keily, R., Astbury, G., & Reith, G. (2014). Risky places?: Mapping gambling machine density and socio-economic deprivation. *Journal of Gambling Studies,* 30, 201–12.

Wardle, H., Moody, A., Spence, S., Orford, J., Volberg, R., Jotangia, D., Griffiths, M., Hussey, D., & Dobbie, F. (2011). *British Gambling Prevalence Survey 2010.* National Centre for Social Research/Gambling Commission. London: The Stationery Office.

Wardle, H., Reith, G., Best, D., McDaid, D., & Platt, S. (2018). Measuring gambling-related harms: a framework for action. Gambling Commission/Responsible Gambling Strategy Board/GambleAware, 2 July 2018.

Wardle, H., Sproston, K., Orford, J., Erens, B., Griffiths, M., Constantine, R., & Pigott, S. (2007). *British Gambling Prevalence Survey 2007.* National Centre for Social Research/Gambling Commission. London: The Stationery Office.

Weatherburn, D. (2009). Dilemmas in harm minimisation. *Addiction,* 104, 335–9.

Weinstock, J. *et al.* (27 others). (2018). Call to action for gambling disorders in the United States. *Addiction,* 113, 1156–58.

Welte, J., Wieczorek, W., Barnes, W., Tidwell, M., & Hoffman, J. (2004). The relationship of ecological and geographic factors to gambling behaviour and pathology. *Journal of Gambling Studies,* 20, 405–23.

Westminster eForum (2012). The UK online gambling industry. Conference held in London, June 2012.

Westminster eForum (2018). Keynote seminar: next steps for the UK gambling industry – innovation, regulation and the future shape of the sector, 18 September 2018.

Wieczorek, Ł, & Bujalski, M. (2018). After the storm: an analysis of gambling legislation in Poland and its effects. In M. Egerer, V. Marionneau, & J. Nikkinen (eds.), *Gambling Policies in European Welfare States: Current Challenges and Future Prospects.* Cham. Switzerland: Palgrave Macmillan, 217–37.

Williams, R., West, B., & Simpson, R. (2007). *Prevention of problem gambling: a comprehensive review of the evidence.* Report prepared for the Ontario problem gambling research centre. Ontario: Guelph.

Williams, R., Wood, R., & Parke, J. (2012). History, current worldwide situation, and concerns with internet gambling. In R. Williams, R. Wood, & J. Parke (eds.), *Routledge International Handbook on Internet Gambling.* London: Routledge (cited by Casey, 2017. 'Getting your money for nothing': narratives of self and value in women's 'at-home' gambling practices. In H. Bowden-Jones & F. Prever (ed.), *Gambling Disorders in Women: An International Female Perspective on Treatment and Research.* London: Routledge, 200–8.).

Wise, R. (2002). Brain reward circuitry: insights from unsensed incentives. *Neuron,* 36, 229–40 (cited by Ross *et al.,* 2008).

Wood, D. (2016). *What Have We Done: The Moral Injury of Our Longest Wars.* New York: Little, Brown & Company.

Wood, R., & Griffiths, M. (2007). A qualitative investigation of problem gambling as an escape-based coping strategy. *Psychology and Psychotherapy: Theory, Research and Practice,* 80, 107–25.

Wood, T., Shorter, G., & Griffiths, M. (2014). Rating the suitability of responsible gambling features for specific game types: a resource for optimizing responsible gambling strategy. *International Journal of Mental Health and Addiction*, 12, 94–112.

World Casino News (2018). Green light given to Phu Quoc casino: locals can gamble there. news.worldcasinodirectory.com, 26 November 2018.

World Health Organisation (2003). *Framework Convention on Tobacco Control*. Geneva: World Health Organization.

World Health Organisation (2010). *Global Strategy to Reduce the Harmful Use of Alcohol*. Geneva: World Health Organization.

World Health Organisation (2018). ICD-11 – Mortality and morbidity statistics international classification of diseases 11th revision. https://icd.who.int.

Wray, M., Miller, M., Gurvey, J., Carroll, J., & Kawachi, I. (2008). Leaving Las Vegas: exposure to Las Vegas and risk of suicide. *Social Science and Medicine*, 67, 1882–8 (cited by Sulkunen *et al.*, 2019).

Yogonet Gaming News (2017a). European Commission green lights gambling expansion in Denmark, 5 June 2017, cited by Global Gambling Guidance group (G4), info@gx4. com, 22 June 2017.

Yogonet Gaming News (2017b). Swiss lawmakers green light online gambling legalization, 12 October 2017, cited by Global Gambling Guidance group (G4), info@gx4.com, 8 November 2017.

Young, M. (2013). Statistics, scapegoats and social control: a critique of pathological gambling prevalence research. *Addiction Research and Theory*, 21, 1–11.

Zinberg, N. (1978). *Drug, Set, and Setting: The Basis for Controlled Intoxicant Use*. New Haven: Yale University Press.

INDEX

Note: **Boldfaced** page references indicate tables. *Italic* references indicate figures.

accessibility of gambling 5, 62, 86–7
acute gambling distress 106
Adams, Peter 39, 44, 49, 56, 130–4, 149
Addiction by Design (Schüll) 74, 88, 134
addiction to gambling: Australian studies of
    94, 99; autonomy and 120; background
    information 90; brain and 103–5; in
    Britain 109; characteristics of 2–3;
    conclusions 107–8; as conditioned
    habit 101–3; conditioning and 102–3;
    conflict and 105–7; dissonance and 106;
    distorted thinking and 95–6; divided
    self and 99–101; electronic gambling
    machines and 80; Finnish study of 94;
    guilt and 99; neuroscience of 103–5;
    Nottingham Trent University study of
    94; overview 2–3, 90, 107; personality
    change and 97–9; person not product
    view of 90; preoccupation and 95, 98;
    recognition of 92–3; reinforcement
    and 102–3; scientific understanding of
    101–7; Scottish study of 100; secrecy and
    97, 100, 116; self-exclusion 90–2; shame
    and 98–9; stories of, real-life 94–101;
    volatility of potential outcome and 103
adult entertainment centres 30
Advertising Association 59
advertising/promotion of gambling: in
    Australia 70–1, 151; Australia's concern
    about children and 70–1; background
    information 58; in Belgium 151–2;
Binde's study on 60–3; British studies
    on 62–4; Canadian study of 63, 65;
    change in, manifesto for **143**, 151–3;
    children and 3, 64–5, 68–72, 139;
    conclusion about 71–2, **71–2**; false
    impression of gambling and 72; 4As
    of starting to gamble and 59; meeting
    pre-existing need view and 58; money
    spent on 59; 9:00 pm TV gambling
    advertising watershed and 138–41;
    of online gambling 62–8; overview
    2; reconsidering 3; Sheffield Hallam
    University study on 63, 85; social
    media and 69–71; sports-related 65–8;
    supply of product effect on gambling
    motivation 58–9; Swedish study on
    60–3; ubiquity of 59–62; whistle to
    whistle ban on 151; winning and, appeal
    and exaggeration of 60–2
Advertising Standards Authority (ASA)
    (Britain) 139–40, 152
Advisory Board for Safer Gambling (ABSG)
    (Britain) 40, 132–3, 146
age restrictions on gambling 22, 160
Ainsworth, Len 28
akrasia 106–7
Albania, resistance to spread of casino
    gambling in 16
alcohol/alcohol industry: addiction
    and 91–3; brain and 104; branch of
    government responsible for 37; divided

self and 100; gambling problems and co-occurrence with dependency on 114; government dependency on 35; harm reduction strategies and 41; harms to others and 110; influence of research experts in 6–7; knowledge chain and 44; policy making and 148; power of 42, 57; unit pricing and, resistance to 154; in venues for gambling, prohibiting 160

All Party Parliamentary Group (APPG) for Betting and Gaming (Britain) 19, 38, 160

ambient gambling (Britain) 7, 162

American Gaming Association (AGA) 53, 131–2

American Psychiatric Association (APA) 92–3, 101

Amusement Caterers' Association 46

Animal Game lottery (Brazil) 16, 33

Anti-Gambling League (Britain) 50

arcades, gambling 30

Aristocratic Leisure gambling company 28

Aristotle 106

Association of British Bookmakers 40–1

Atherton, Mike 19

Atlantic City (USA) gambling venue 115

attributable fraction 112

Australia: accessibility of gambling study in 86–7; addiction to gambling studies in 94, 99; advertising/promotion of gambling in 70–1, 151; cost-benefit analysis of gambling in 120; dependence on gambling **36**; electronic gambling machines **7**, 8–9, 15, 43, 121; financial problems study, gambling-related 116; gambling industry in 5; gambling as part of heritage and 49; harms of gambling studies in 110, 116–18, 122–3; Ladbrokes Card in 70; market for gambling in 26; Melbourne study in 86–7; monopolies in 33; normalisation of gambling in 123; Office of Film and Literature Classification 12; online gambling in 12, **13**; personal responsibility discourse and 51; relationship problems study in, gambling-related 117–18; Royal Commission on Gambling 6; self-exclusion in 91; suburban gambling in 7, 121; Victorian Responsible Gambling Foundation 57; voluntary pre-commitment in 8; warnings about Big Gambling and 38; Yalata Aboriginal community in 122–3

Australian Gambling Council 46

Australian Gaming Machine Manufacturers Association 48

Australian Productivity Commission 120, 150

Austria, electronic gambling machines in 33; *see also* Casinos Austria

autonomy and addiction to gambling 120

Babor, Tom 132

backlash against gambling: attitudes that gambling is dangerous 24; children and, intensification of concern about 21–3; citizens' voices 23–4; electronic gambling machines and 6–9, **7**; Fixed Odds Betting Terminals and 18–21; gambling industry and, questions about responses to 30–1; growing 24–5; liberalisation of gambling and 1, 17–18; start of 1

bankruptcy, gambling-related 112–13

Belgium: advertising/promotion of gambling in 151–2; online gambling in 12, **13**

Bergmo, Lill-Tove 8

Berridge, K. 104

bet365 gambling company 27, 67

betting 27, 84–5; *see also* sports betting

betting exchanges 9

Betting, Lotteries, and Gaming Royal Commission (Britain) 6, 46

Betting Their Lives (Tepperman) 117

Bikini Poker 64

Binde, Per 60–3, 139–40, 153

bingo game 14, 17, 17–18, 22, 87

Blair, Tony 18

blaming the victim 53

Blaszczynski, Alex 131, 136

Boateng, Paul 48

Boyd Law School (University of Nevada) 132

Brady, Maggie 123

brain and addiction 103–5

Brazil: Animal Game lottery in 16, 33; pressure to expand gambling in 16–17

Britain: accessibility to gambling study in 87; addiction to gambling in 109; advertising/promotion of gambling studies in 62–4; Advertising Standards Authority 139–40, 152; Advisory Board for Safer Gambling 40, 132–3, 146; All Party Parliamentary Group for Betting and Gaming 19, 38, 160; ambient gambling in 7, 162; Amusement Caterers' Association 46; Anti-Gambling League 50; Association of British Bookmakers 40–1; branches of government responsible for gambling in 37; Broadcast Committee of Advertising Practice 38,

139–41; case studies of research and Gambling Establishment 135–41; Centre for Evidence and Policy 128; Code of Advertising Practice 69; Committee of Advertising Practice 38, 69, 139–41, 152; Conservative Government in 1; demand test and 17–18, 121; Department for Digital, Culture, Media and Sports 22, 29–30, 37, 46, 91, 147; Department of Health 37, 147; dependence on gambling and 35–6, **36**; electronic gambling machines in 8, 19, 22, 29, 121–2; Fairer Gambling Campaign 19, 147; family entertainment centres in 122; Fixed Odds Betting Terminals in 8, 29, 48, 51, 135–8, 146, 160; football in 66–8; football pools in 1930s 73–4, 77, 88; GambleAware 40–1, 57, 132–3, 156; Gambling Act (2005) 1, 18, 20, 59, 91, 121, 126, 138, 140, 142, 144, 149, 162; Gambling Commission 10, 19–20, 34, 40–1, 91, 109, 133, 139, 146, 151, 156–7; Gambling Establishment 40, *40*; gambling industry in 5; Gambling with Lives 23–4, 115; gambling machines research project in 135–8; Gambling Review Body 18, 22, 37, 47, 126, 160, 162; Gambling Watch UK 23, 94–5, 98, 118, 138; health policy of, influence on 42; homelessness study in, gambling-related 113; Home Office 37; inequality study in, gambling-related 124–5; Labour Government in 1, 18, 20, 129, 142, 147; liberalisation of gambling in 17–18; Lottery Commission 125; Machines Research Oversight Panel 136–7; Manchester United Poker 64; market for gambling in 27; mega-casino complexes in 18; National Health Service-based system of treatment for gambling problems 4, 121, 163–4; National Housing and Town Planning Council report (1988) 22; National Lottery Act (1993) 17; National Lottery in 32, 125, 150, 160; Next Steps for the UK Gambling Industry conference (2018) 30–1; 9:00 pm TV gambling advertising watershed 138–41; Nottingham Trent studies in 62, 64, 87, 94; online gambling in 29; point-of-consumption tax in 34; Portman Group 41; prevention, treatment and research of gambling in, funding 150; public attitude surveys on gambling in 24, 87, 124, 150; Public Health Responsibility Deal 42; regulation of gambling in 34; Responsible Gambling Fund 41; Responsible Gambling Strategy Board 51–2, 132–3, 146, 162–3; Responsible Gambling Trust 40–1, 51, 57, 132, 135, 157; Royal Commission on Betting, Lotteries, and Gaming 6, 46; self-exclusion in 91; surveys on gambling in 24; *see also specific law*
British Advertising Standards Authority 70
British Amusement Catering Trade Association (BACTA) 30
British Beer and Pub Association 30
British Gambling Prevalence Survey (2007) 24
British Gambling Prevalence Survey (2010) 24, 116, 150
British-Spanish collaborative research group 68
Broadcast Committee of Advertising Practice (BCAP) (Britain) 38, 139–41
Brown, Gordon 18
Budd, Sir Alan 20
business as usual discourse *44*, 47–8, 144

Cake Poker 63
Cameron, David 43
Campaign for Fairer Gambling (Britain) 19, 147
Canada: advertising/promotion of gambling study in 63, 65; arousal of gamblers during play study in 85; deception of gamblers study in 88; dependence on gambling **36**; Fixed Odds Betting Terminals study in 148; harms approach to gambling in 109; market for gambling in 27; payback percentage study in 78–9; Probability Accounting Report sheets for slot machines in 78; relationship problems study in, gambling-related 117; self-exclusion in 91; volatility in potential outcome study in 76–8
Canadian Freedom of Information and Protection of Privacy Act 78
Cardano, Jerome 92
Casey, D. 17
casino gambling: floating offshore 15; resistance to spread of 14–16, 48
Casinos Austria 28, 33
Centre for Evidence and Policy (Britain) 128
Centre for the Study of Gambling (University of Salford, England) 46
chances of winning, deception about 88–9
change, manifesto for: advertising/ promotion of gambling issues **143**,

151–3; ambient gambling reduction 162; background information 142; comprehensive treatment of problem gamblers **144**, 162–5; conclusions 165–6; cross-department issue in government 3, 147; dangerous consumption/public health perspective 3, 145; gambling harm prevention, funding 149–50; gambling prevention, funding 147–50; government's role, rethinking 142, **143**; impact assessment of gambling 161–2; national government strategy for gambling, need for 142, 146; national strategy with government 3, 146–7; ordinary business/responsible gambling ideology 3, 144; overview 3–4, 142, **143**; policymaking 147–50; *see also* harm reduction (HR) strategies

Chan, Margaret 148

charitable donations by gambling industry 49–50

children: advertising/promotion of gambling and 3, 64–5, 68–72, 139; age restrictions on gambling and 22, 160; backlash against gambling and intensification of concern about 21–3; education about gambling for 163–4; harms of gambling to 119–20; online gambling and, dangers of 10–11

China, resistance to spread of casino gambling in 15

Citizens Against Gambling (Czech Republic) 8

citizens' voices in backlash against gambling 23–4

Clark, Luke 148

Clubs Australia 49

ClubsNSW 8

Coates, Denise 28

Code of Advertising Practice (Britain) 69

cognitive behaviour therapy (CBT) 163

'cognitive capture' 43

Collins, Peter 46, 50

Committee of Advertising Practice (CAP) (Britain) 38, 69, 139–41, 152

community harms of gambling **111**, 120–3

complex bets 85

conditioned habit, addiction as 101–3

conditioned stimulus (CS) 103

conditioning perspective 102–3

conflict and addiction to gambling 105–7

control in gambling, illusion of 84–5

co-occurrence or problems 114–15, 118, 163

coping dilemmas 116–17

crime, gambling-related 113–14

Crouch, Tracey 8

Crown-Bet online gambling company 28

cultural/social benefits discourse *44*, 48–50

Czech Republic: Citizens Against Gambling 8; electronic gambling machines in 7–8, **7**

da Cunha, Derek 16

dangerousness of gambling 24, 145

Danske Spil gambling company 14

Davies, Philip 38

debt, gambling-related 112–13

deception of gamblers: addiction by design 74–6; Canadian study of 88; chances of winning 88–9; complex bets 84; conclusions 88–9; illusion of skill/control 84–5; in-play bets 84; losses disguised as wins 82–4; motivation for gambling and 73; music as distraction 86; near misses 84; odds of winning 80–5; online sports gamblers 80–5; overview 2–3, 73–4; payback percentage information, misleading/irrelevant 78–80; skewed distributions of wins 79–80; venues for gambling and 85–7; volatility in potential outcome disguising operator's advantage 76–8

demand test 17–18, 121

Denmark: branch of government responsible for gambling in 38; monopolies in 14, 32; online gambling in 14

Department for Digital, Culture, Media and Sports (DCMS) (Britain) 22, 29–30, 37, 46, 91, 147

Department of Health (Britain) 37, 141

dependence on gambling: by governments 35–6, **36**; by other parties 38–9

depoliticisation process 129

Designing Casinos to Dominate the Competition (Friedman) 86

Dewey, John 102

Diagnostic and Statistical Manual (DSM) 93

discourse on gambling *see* Establishment discourse

dissonance and addiction to gambling 106

distorted thinking and addiction to gambling 95–6

distributions of wins, skewed 79–80, 134

divided self and addiction to gambling 99–101

Dixon, Mike 78–9

domestic abuse, gambling-related 118

dopamine system 106–7
Dostoevsky, F. 103
dual-process decision theory 107

education about gambling 154–5, 163–4
e-help for gambling problems 164
electronic gambling machines (EGMs):
  addiction to gambling and 80; in
  Australia **7**, 8–9, 15, 43, 121; in Austria
  33; backlash against 6–9, **7**; in Britain 8,
  19, 22, 29–30, 84–5, 121–2; in Czech
  Republic 7–8, **7**; in France 9; harmless
  entertainment discourse and 46; in Italy
  7, **7**; in Las Vegas 52; in Norway **7**, 8; in
  Nova Scotia 160; in Poland **7**; regulation
  of 7–8, **7**, 46; in Russia **7**; transformation
  caused by 74–5; types of 75; volatility in
  potential outcome and 76–8
employment problems, gambling-related
  113–14
Entertainment Software Rating Board
  (USA) 12
Establishment discourse: background
  information 42–4; blaming the
  victim and 53; challenging, need for
  56–7; elements, overview 2, 44, *44*;
  freedom to choose *44*, 50–1; harmless
  entertainment 44–7, *44*, 53–4, 73, 145;
  interests of gambling industry and 44,
  53–6; ordinary business *44*, 47–8, 144;
  overview 2; personal responsibility *44*,
  51–3, 54–6; power of gambling industry
  and 42–4; social/cultural benefits *44*,
  48–50; studies examining 53–6
*Establishment and How They Get Away With
  It, The* (Jones) 43
European Court of Justice 34
European Union 34–5, 145; *see also specific
  country*
evidence-based policy 128–9

Fable 2 game 12
Facebook 69–70
Fairer Gambling Campaign (Britain) 19,
  147
Fair Game report 130
false impression of gambling in advertising 72
Families Against Casinos (Singapore) 15
family entertainment centres 122
family harms of gambling **111**, 115–20
FanDuel gambling company 31
fantasy sports betting 10
Featurespace research organisation 137
FIFA Ultimate Team game 11–12

financial counseling 163–4
financial problems, gambling-related
  112–13, 116–17
Finland: addiction to gambling study in
  94; branch of government responsible
  for gambling 38; branch of government
  responsible for gambling in 38;
  dependence on gambling **36**; mandatory
  limits in 158; market for gambling in 27;
  monopolies in 32; University of Helsinki
  recommendations 145; Veikkus RAY
  model 32, 161
5-Step Method 165
Five Play, Ten Play game 75
Fixed Odds Betting Terminals (FOBTs
  or fob-tees): backlash against gambling
  and 18–21; in Britain 8, 29, 48, 51,
  135–8, 146, 160; Canadian study of 148;
  defending 161–2; lessons of, learning
  161
football in Britain 66–8
football pools in 1930s (Britain) 73–4, 77,
  88
Forza Motorsport 7 game 12
4As of starting to gamble 59
France: dependence on gambling by **36**;
  electronic gambling machines in 9;
  online gambling in **13**
free bets offer 62, 140, 151
freedom to choose discourse *44*, 50–1
free trade rules (European Union) 34

Gainsbury, Sally 10–11
GambleAware (Britain) 40–1, 57, 132–3,
  156
Gambler, The (Dostoevsky) 103
Gambling (Atherton) 19
Gambling Act (2005) (Britain) 1, 18, 20, 59,
  91, 121, 126, 138, 140, 142, 144, 149, 162
Gambling Commission (GC) (Britain) 10,
  19–20, 34, 40–1, 91, 109, 133, 139, 146,
  151, 156–7
Gambling Establishment: British 40, *40*;
  conclusions about 39–41; defining 1, 26,
  39–40; gambling education and 154–5;
  gambling industry 26–32; governments
  32–8; harm reduction strategies and 153,
  157–8; new thinking about, need for
  3, 57, 142, 144–7; other partners 38–9;
  overview 1–2, 26; power of 5, 25, 166;
  research agenda on gambling and 42; *see
  also* Establishment discourse; gambling
  industry; research and Gambling
  Establishment

gambling evidence-policy link 128–30
gambling fever 106
gambling-habit development 101–3
gambling industry: aspirations of 28–32;
in Australia 5; in Britain 5; casinos and,
resistance to spread of 14–16; charitable
donations by 49–50; consolidation in
28; current climate 1; Establishment
discourse and interests of 44, 53–6;
expansion of 1, 5–6, 16–17; gross
gambling revenue 26–8, 35; harm
reduction strategies and, ambivalence
about 153–4; knowledge chain and 44;
liberalisation and 1, 14, 17–18, 126;
lobbying by 42–3; market growth in
27; monopolies 14, 32; in Poland 5;
power of 42–4; in South Africa 50–1;
transformation of 5–6; in USA 6, 28;
world market 26–7; *see also* backlash
against gambling; electronic gambling
machines (EGMs); online gambling
Gambling with Lives (GwL) (Britain)
23–4, 115
gambling machines research project
(Britain) 135–8
Gambling Prevalence Survey (2007)
(Britain) 24
Gambling Prevalence Survey (2010)
(Britain) 24, 116, 150
gambling problems *see* harms of gambling
Gambling and the Public Interest (Collins) 50
Gambling Review Body (GRB) (Britain) 18,
22, 37, 47, 126, 160, 162
gambling-sports link 11, 65–8
*Gambling Threat to National and Homeland
Security, The,* report (2012) (USA) 132
Gambling Watch UK (GWUK) 23, 94–5,
98, 118, 138
GamStop 9, 157
geo-temporal accessibility 86
Germany: dependence on gambling **36**;
illegal gambling in 33; inequality study
in, gambling-related 124; mandatory
limits in 158; market for gambling,
potential 31–2; online gambling in 12, **13**
Gillard, Julia 8
Goldsmiths conference (2014) (London) 130
good life for all, gambling's harm to 126–7
Goodwin, B. 116
governments: branches responsible for
gambling 37–8, 147; gambling as cross-
department issue and 3, 147; Gambling
Establishment and 32–8; regulation of
gambling by 34–5; *see also specific country*

Grand Theft Auto game 12
Great Britain *see* Britain
Griffiths, Mark 10, 68, 84, 132
gross gambling revenue (GGR) 26, 26–8, 35
Gross Gambling Yield (GGY) 149–50
Grout, Gardner 76
guilt and addiction to gambling 99

habit: addiction to gambling as conditioned
101–3; moral 106–7
Hamann, Dietmar 67
Hancock, L. 46, 51
harmless entertainment discourse 44–7, *44*,
53–4, 73, 145
harmonisation of gambling regulation 29,
145
harm reduction (HR) strategies: age
restrictions on gambling 160; alcohol
industry and 41; ambivalence about, by
gambling industry 153–4; challenging
Gambling Establishment 158–60;
core idea of 153; education about
gambling 154–5; evaluative research
on 159; funding 149–50; Gambling
Establishment 153, 157–8; rethinking
3; reviewing effectiveness of 159; *Setting
Limits* report (2018) and 159; stronger
forms of, to challenge Gambling
Establishment 158–60; tracking/
identifying problem gamblers 155–7; *see
also* change, manifesto for
harms approach to gambling 109, 127; *see
also* harms of gambling
harms of gambling: attributable fraction and
112; Australian studies of 110, 116–18,
122–3; background information 109–10;
bankruptcy 112–13; to children 119–20;
to communities **111**, 120–3; conclusions
127; crime 113–14; debt 112–13;
domestic abuse 118; employment
problems 113–14; to family members
of gamblers **111**, 115–20; financial
problems 112–13, 116–17; to gamblers
111, 112–15; good life for all and,
endangering 126–7; health problems
118–19; homelessness 113; inequality
124–5; job loss 113–14; main areas,
summary of 110, **111**, 112; *Measuring
gambling-related harms* report (2018)
110; mental health problems 114–15;
overview 3, 109, 127; press reaction to 8;
prevention paradox and 112; relationship
problems 117–18; to society **111**, 123–7;
substance use disorders 114–15; suicide

115; trust, loss of 117; work problems 113–14; *see also* harm reduction (HR) theory
harms to others (HtO) 110
Harrigan, Kevin 78–9
Harvard Medical School studies on gamblers 80–2, 134
Hattersley, Lord 126–7
health problems, gambling-related 118–19
Heather, Nick 107
helplines for gambling problems 164
homelessness, gambling-related 113
Home Office (Britain) 37
Hong Kong, dependency on gambling by 39
horse race betting 10, 14, 16, 32, 37, 50, 67, 87, 122
How Much Is Enough? (Skidelsky and Skidelsky) 126
Hundred Play Poker game 75

identifying problem gamblers 155–7
illegal gambling 33–4
illusion of gambling skill/control 84–5
impact assessment of gambling 161–2
India: casino gambling in, resistance to spread of 15; illegal gambling in 33–4
inequality, gambling-related 124–5
'informed consumers' 52
in-play betting 65, 84
Institute for Public Policy Research (IPPR) 110, 124, 146–7
Institute for Research on Gambling (IRG) (Harvard) 131–2
International Charter for Gambling 145
International Classification of Diseases 93
International Gaming Research Unit (Nottingham Trent University, Britain) 62, 94, 132
International Lottery (Liechtenstein) 9
internet gambling *see* online gambling
Ireland, market for gambling in 26–7
Islamic countries, pressure to expand gambling in 17
Italy: dependence on gambling in **36**; electronic gambling machines in **7**; market for gambling in 27; No Slot Movement in 8

James, William 102, 106
Japan, resistance to spread of casino gambling in 16
job loss, gambling-related 113–14
Jones, Carwyn 67, 69
Jones, Owen 43–4

Karolinska University Hospital (Sweden) 55
Karter, Liz 94–6, 98, 101
Kelly, Tony 94, 96–7, 99–100, 103, 113
King, D. 12
'knowledge chain' 44

Ladbrokes gambling company 28, 31, 70
land-based gambling/operators 9, 28, 31, 156, 162
Larcombe, Justyn 94–8, 99–101
Las Vegas (USA) gambling venue 28, 52, 74–6
Las Vegas effect 115
Learning from Las Vegas (Venturi and colleagues) 86
Lee Kuan Yew 14, 16
legacy effects 110, 117
Legacy Tobacco Documents Library 148
legislation *see* regulation of gambling; *specific law*
Levy, N. 105
Lewis, Marc 102
liberalisation of gambling/gambling industry 1, 14, 17–18, 126
Lions Foundation 49–50
live-action sports betting 65
Livingstone, Charles 43, 47, 131
loan sharks 116
loot boxes 11–12
Lopez-Gonzalez, H. 68, 84
losses disguised as wins (LDWs) 2, 74, 82–4
loss limits, voluntary 157–8
lotteries 9, 27, 32–3, 34, 49, 61; *see also specific name*
Lottery Commission (Britain) 125
loyalty cards 54, 136
Lucky Larry's Lobstermania game machine 78

Macau, resistance to spread of casino gambling in 15
Machines Research Oversight Panel (Britain) 136–7
Malaysia, pressure to expand gambling in 17
Manchester United Poker (Britain) 64
mandatory limits 158
markets for gambling 26–7, 31–2, 35
Mass Observation research organisation 73–4, 77, 88
Match of the Day (BBC programme) 67–8, 151
Measuring gambling-related harms report (2018) 110
mega-casino complexes 18

mental health problems, gambling related
114–15
Miers, David 21–2
Mill, John Stuart 51
monetisation schemes, predatory 11–12
monitoring system, interactive 55
monopolies 14, 32–3
moral habits 106–7
Moral Jeopardy (Adams) 39, 44, 131
motivational interviewing (MI) 163
motivation for gambling 58–9, 63, 73
music as distraction 86

Nasty Duck gambling activity 64–5
NatCen research organisation 137
National Association for Gambling Addicts
(SBRF) (Sweden) 55
National Center for Responsible Gaming
(NCRG) 131–2, 134
National Health Service-based system of
treatment for gambling problems 4, 121,
163–4
National Housing and Town Planning
Council report (1988) (Britain) 22
National Lottery (Britain) 32, 125, 150, 160
National Lottery Act (1993) (Britain) 17
National Opinion Poll survey (2003) 24
National Problem Gambling Clinic
(Britain) 39, 121, 165
nature of gambling 45
near misses 84
Netherlands, market for gambling in 31–2
neuroscience of addiction to gambling
103–5
New Jersey (USA), market for gambling
in 35
New Zealand: harms approach to gambling
in 109; inequality study in, gambling
related 125; market for gambling in 27;
motivation for gambling study in 59;
personal responsibility discourse and 51;
self-exclusion in 91
Next Steps for the UK Gambling Industry
conference (2018) (Britain) 30–1
9:00 pm TV gambling advertising
watershed 138–41
non-monetary forms of gambling 12
normalisation of gambling 10, 63, 123–4, 140
Norsk Tipping (Norwegian state-owned
company) 38, 83
North African countries, pressure to expand
gambling in 17
Norway: branch of government responsible
for gambling in 38; dependence on

gambling **36**; electronic gambling
machines in **7**, 8; losses disguised as wins
study in 83; market for gambling in 27;
online gambling in 34; press reaction to
harm of gambling 8
No Slot Movement (Italy) 8
Nottingham Trent studies (Britain) 62, 64,
87, 94
Nova Scotia, electronic gambling machines
in 160
Novomatic Group gambling company 28

odds of winning, deception of gamblers and
80–5
Ofcom 59, 68
Office of Film and Literature Classification
(Australia) 12
offshore gambling 15, 35
online gambling: accessibility to gambling
and 87–8; advertising/promotion of
62–8; in Australia 12, **13**; in Belgium
13; bingo 17; in Britain 29; children and,
dangers of 10–11; deception of sports
gamblers and 80–5; in Denmark 14;
establishment of 9; forms of gambling
9–10; in France **13**; games 11–12; in
Germany 12, **13**; gross gambling revenue
and 27–8; growth of 27; harmonisation
of regulation of gambling, call for 29;
lotteries 34; monopolies 14; in Norway
34; offshore 35; regulation 12, **13**, 14, 29;
social media and 11–12; sports 80–2;
in Sweden **13**, 14; in Switzerland **13**; in
USA 12, **13**, 35
Ontario Problem Gambling Research
Centre 117
ordinary business discourse *44*, 47–8, 144
Osborne, George 28
Österreichische Lotterien (Austria) 33

Packer, James 28
Paddy Power Betfair gambling company 9,
27, 31, 70, 84
Palladium Lounge Status 64
Party Poker 63–4
pathological gambling 92–3
Pavlov, Ivan 103
payback percentage information,
misleading/irrelevant 78–80
personality change and addiction to
gambling 97–9
personal responsibility discourse *44*, 51–3,
54–6
Playscan (interactive monitoring service) 55

point-of-consumption tax 34
Poker Joint 65
Poker Stars 63
poker tournaments 9, 63–5
Poland: electronic gambling machines in **7**;
    gambling industry in 5
policy-based evidence 128, 130
policy-gambling evidence link 128–30
policymaking/policymakers, gambling
    42–4, 147–50; *see also* regulation of
    gambling
Portman Group (Britain) 41
Portugal, regulation of gambling in 34
post-reinforcement pause 83
preoccupation and addiction to gambling
    95, 98
prevention paradox 112
prevention, treatment and research (PT&R)
    of gambling, funding 149–50
Pricewaterhouse Coopers (PwC) report 30
Probability Accounting Report (PAR)
    sheets for slot machines 78
problem gambling 53, 114, 126, 155–7; *see
    also* harms of gambling; treatment for
    gambling problems
Problem Gambling Severity Index 136, 156
prohibition of gambling 24, 50
Project Entropia game 11
promotion of gambling *see* advertising/
    promotion of gambling
public health model 45
Public Health Responsibility Deal
    (Britain) 42

random reinforcement (RR) 103
RAY (Finland's Slot Machine Association)
    32, 161
Recommendations on Principles for the
    Protection of Consumers and Players of
    Online Gambling and for the Prevention
    of Minors from Gambling Online
    (European Commission) 69
Red Card (Kelly) 94
regulation of gambling: in Britain 34;
    'cognitive capture' and 43; demand test
    17–18; electronic gambling machines
    7–8, **7**, 46; European Union rules 34–5;
    by governments 34–5; harmonisation
    of, call for 29, 145; historic perspective
    of 14; local 162; online gambling 12,
    13, 14, 29; in Portugal 34; 'regulatory
    pyramid' and 162; in USA 31, 35; World
    Trade Organisation rules 34–5; *see also
    specific law*

reinforcement and addiction to gambling
    102–3
relationship problems, gambling-related
    117–18
remote gambling *see* online gambling
Reno model of gambling 45–6, 50–2, 131,
    158
research and Gambling Establishment:
    British case studies 135–41; conclusions
    141; criticisms of 130–41; funding
    and lack of independence 130–3;
    gambling evidence-policy link and
    128–30; gambling machines research
    project 135–8; influence on content of
    research 133–4; 9:00 pm TV gambling
    advertising watershed 138–41; overview
    3, 141
resisting power of Gambling Establishment
    see change, manifesto for
responsibility services 54
'responsible gambling' 51–4, 153
Responsible Gambling Fund (Britain) 41
Responsible Gambling Strategy Board (now
    Advisory Board for Safer Gambling)
    (Britain) 51–2, 132–3, 146, 162–3
Responsible Gambling Trust (RGT) (now
    GambleAware) (Britain) 40–1, 51, 57,
    132, 135, 157
return to player (RTP) 78–81, *82*
reward conditioning 102
risk society, development of 126
Robinson, T. 104
Rockem Poker gambling activity 64
Room, Robin 131
'roulette machines' *see* Fixed Odds Betting
    Terminals (FOBTs)
Rowe, Bruce 76
Royal Commission on Betting, Lotteries,
    and Gaming (Britain) 6, 46
Royal Commission on Gambling
    (Australia) 6
Rudd, Kevin 8
Russia, electronic gambling machines in **7**

Safe Bet for Success, A (British document) 47
Savage, Robbie 67
schedule of reinforcement 102–3
Schüll, Natasha 52–3, 74–6, 86, 88, 134
Scottish study of addiction to gambling 100
secrecy and addiction to gambling 97,
    100, 116
self-control 157–8; *see also* self-exclusion
self-exclusion 90–2, 157–8
Senet group 151

Setting Limits review (2018) 159
Shaffer, Howard 131–2
shame and addiction to gambling 98–9
Sheffield Hallam University study (Britain) 63, 85
Singapore: casino gambling in, resistance to spread of 14–16; Families Against Casinos 15; financial problems study, gambling-related 116; market for gambling in 26
Singapore Places Its Bets (da Cunha) 16
Singer, Merrill 57
skewed distribution of wins 79–80, 134
Skidelsky, E. 126
Skildelsky, R. 126
skill, illusion of gambling 84–5
Skinner, B F 84, 102–3
Sky Bet Championship 67
Sky Betting & Gaming company 28
Smith, G. 46, 51
Social Aspects and Public Relations Organisation (SAPRO) 41
social/cultural benefits discourse *44*, 48–50
social media: advertising/promotion of gambling and 69–71; online gambling and 11–12
social media; *see also specific name*
social/personal accessibility 86–7
society harms of gambling **111**, 123–7
South Africa: casino gambling in, resistance to spread of 15–16, 48; commission report 49; gambling industry in 50–1; personal responsibility discourse and 50–1
Spain: branch of government responsible for gambling in 37; in-play betting in 84
Spin Poker 75
sports betting 5, 9, 31, 65–8, 84
sports-gambling link 11, 65–8
sports-related advertising/promotion of gambling 65–8
spread betting 9–10
stand-alone gambling games 12
Stars Group company 28
Star Wars: Battlefront II 11
Stiglitz, Joseph 43
Stockholm Addiction Treatment Centre 55
stock market betting 9–10
Stringman, Chris 94–7, 113
substance use disorders 91, 93, 114–15
suburban gambling (Australia) 7, 121
suicide, gambling-related 115
Sulkunen, P. 28, 33, 35–6, 112, 124–5
Svenska Spel company 14, 54–5, 60

Sweden: advertising/promotion of gambling study in 60–3; dependence on gambling and **36**; Karolinska University Hospital 55; market for gambling, potential 31; online gambling in **13**, 14; personal responsibility and gambling 55–6; suicide risk study in, gambling-related 115
Switzerland: online gambling in **13**; self-exclusion in 90; tracking/identifying problem gamblers study in 155

Tails I Lose (Larcombe) 94
telescoping behavior 94
Thatcher, Margaret 17
32Red case 21
time limits 158
time-outs 157–8
tobacco/tobacco industry 35, 114, 133, 148, 160
total consumption theory 45
tracking problem gamblers 155–7
treatment for gambling problems: cognitive behaviour therapy 163; comprehensive 4, **144**, 162–5; effective 164; e-help 164; family's role in 164–5; financial counseling 163–4; 5-Step Method 165; funding 149–50; gambling education 163–4; 'gap' in 163; location of 163; motivational interviewing 163; National Health Service-based system of 4, 121, 163–4; National Problem Gambling Clinic (London) 39, 121, 165; Triangle Approach and 164–5; type of 163; *see also* harm reduction (HR) strategies
Triangle Approach to treatment for gambling problems 164–5
Triple Play Draw Poker 75
trust, gambling and loss of 117
Turner, Nigel 77
24-hour gambling 5, 62, 87–8; *see also* online gambling
Twitter 69–70

United Kingdom *see* Britain
University of Helsinki (Finland) 145
Unlawful Internet Gambling Enforcement Act (UIGEA) (USA) 10, 35
USA: Atlantic City gambling venue 115; bankruptcy-filing rates in 113; casino gambling in, spread of 15; dependence on gambling 35–6, **36**; Entertainment Software Rating Board 12; gambling industry in 6, 28; *Gambling Threat to*

National and Homeland Security report 132; illegal gambling in 33; inequality study in, gambling-related 125; Las Vegas gambling venue 28, 52, 74–6, 115; market for gambling in 27; New Jersey market for gambling 35, 115; offshore gambling and 35; online gambling in 12, **13**, 35; regulation of gambling in 31, 35; Unlawful Internet Gambling Enforcement Act 10, 35

variable reward (VR) 103
Veikkaus RAY model 32, 161
Veikkaus's monopoly 32
Venturi, R. 86
venues for gambling: accessibility of 86; alcohol in, prohibiting 160; arcades 3; attractiveness of 87; deception of gamblers and 85–7; designs of 86; door-to-door transportation to 86; locations of 86; local people and 16; mega-casino complexes 18; safety of 87; *see also specific name/type*
Victorian Responsible Gambling Foundation (VRGF) (Australia) 57
Video Lottery Terminals 33
video poker 75
Vietnam, resistance to spread of casino gambling in 15
volatility in potential outcome 76–8, 103

voluntary loss limits 157–8
voluntary pre-commitment 8

Wardle, Heather 87
whistle to whistle ban on advertising/promotion of gambling 151
William Hill gambling company 21, 27–8, 31, 59–60
Wilson, Joelson 137
Win2Day gambling company 28
Win, Lose, Repeat (Stringman) 94
winning: appeal of, exaggeration of 60–2; chances of, deception about 88–9; losses disguised as wins and 2, 74, 82–4; as motivation for gambling 63, 73; odds of, deception about 80–5
Winstone, Ray 67
women and gambling 87, 94, 100, 125
Women and Problem Gambling (Karter) 94
Woolley, Richard 43, 47
work problems, gambling-related 113–14
World Health Organisation (WHO) 93, 101, 110, 145, 148, 162
World Trade Organisation (WTO) 34–5
World of Warcraft game 11
Wynn, Steve 86

Yalat Aboriginal community (Australia) 122–3
Young, Martin 134
young people/youth *see* children

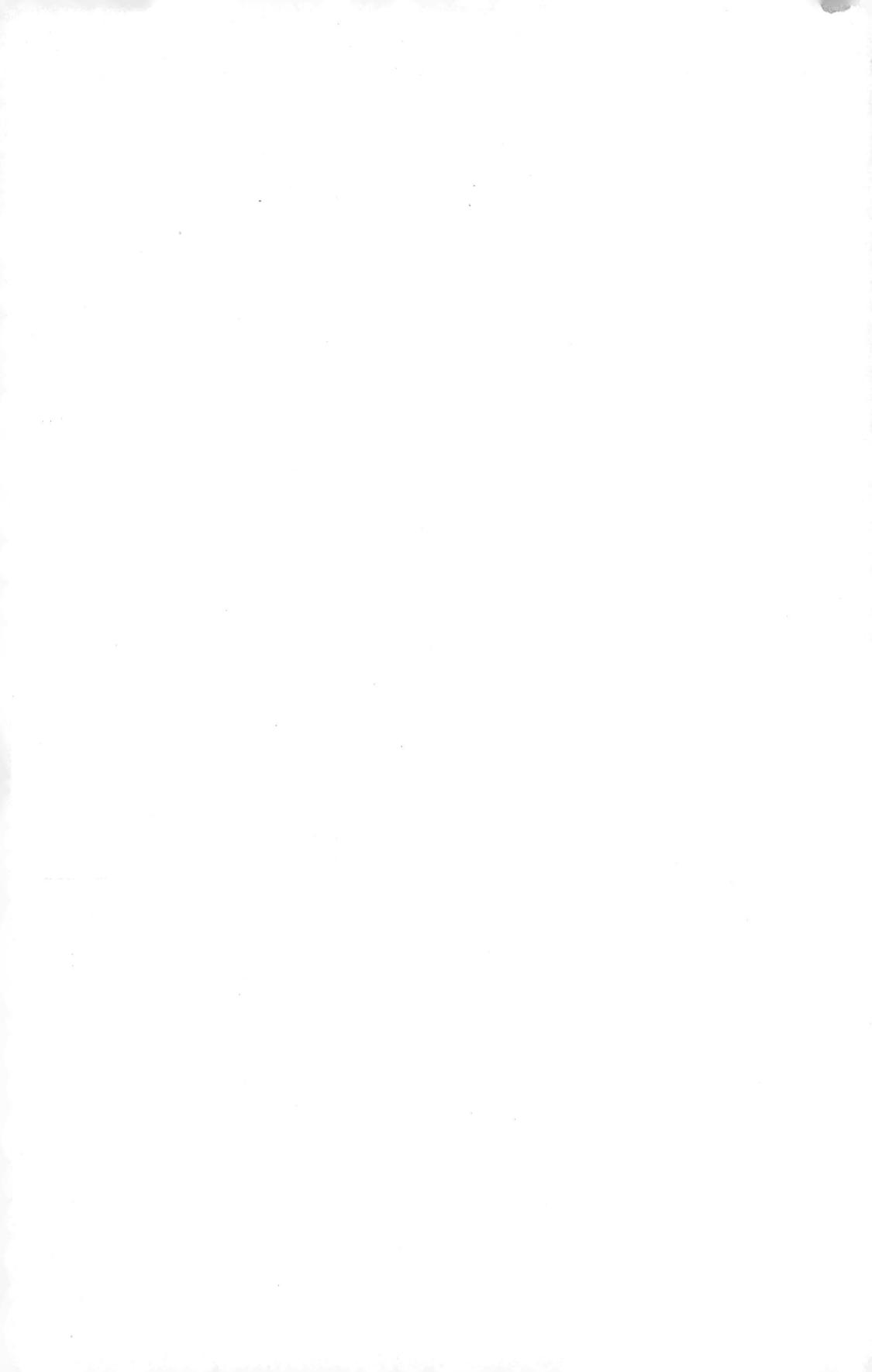

Printed in Great Britain
by Amazon